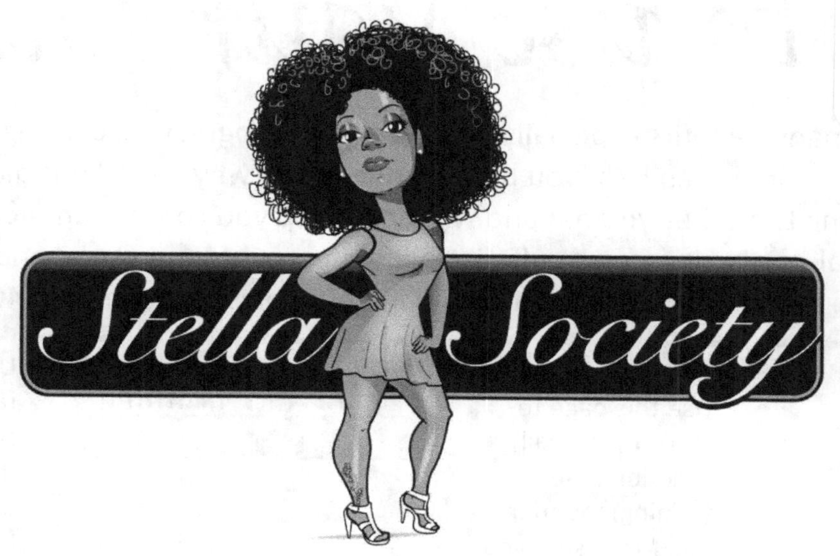

Thank you for participating in the Stella Project 2.0, a 40 day fitness confidence and nutrition challenge. If you purchased this journal and you are not a member of the Stella Project, no worries. You can find us at stellasocietyacademy dot com, or just use it on your own 40 day fitness journey.

Always consult a physician before beginning an exercise program.

How to use your journal

Journaling has many benefits especially when tracking progress. Recording your thoughts before training can help you better understand why a workout did or didn't go too well. Recalling the times you eat and what can help you combat unnecessary cravings. Journaling also increases self-discipline, improves your mood and boost comprehension. Please use this journal to aid in your goals through your 40 days.

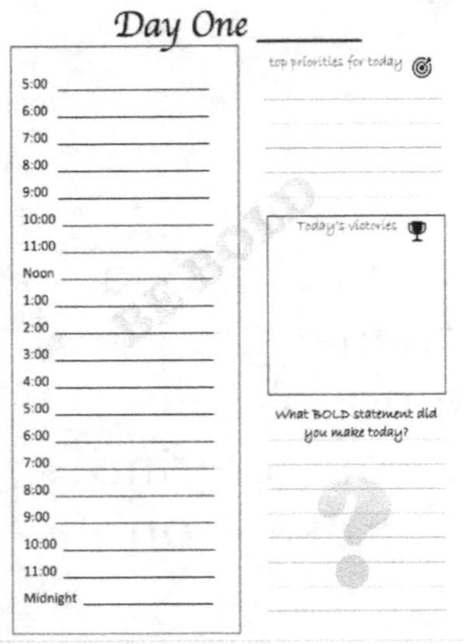

Use this page to record your daily schedule, meals, training, meetings, etc. Make sure you put the date. List your top priorities hat must be completed that day. Record your victories, like drinking all your water and reflect on the daily bestellatude

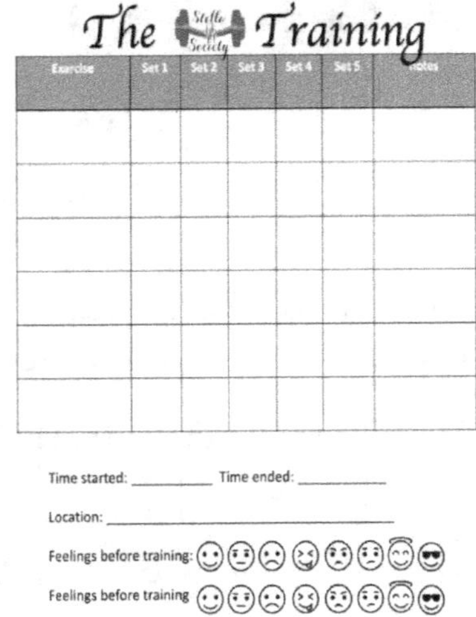

Use this page to record your training sessions. Write them down ahead of time and watch the video in case you have questions. Put the time your started and completed the training as well as how you felt before and after. Leave a note as to why you felt a certain before the training. This could effect how it went.

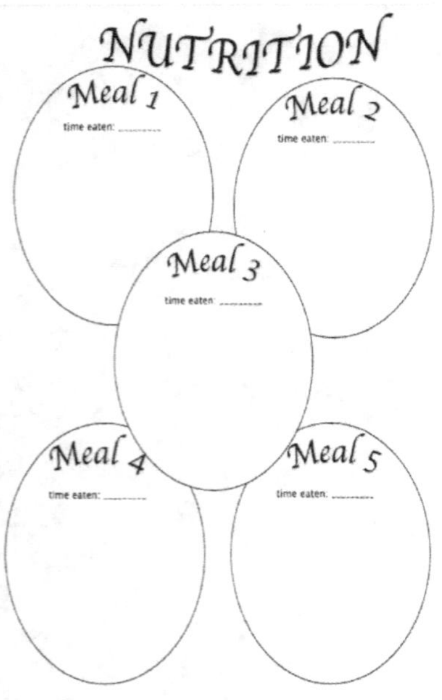

Use this page to record your meals and the time you ate them. This is important especially when tracking your progress. Try to eat your meals at the same time each day. Get your machine on a schedule so it knows how to operate its fuel.

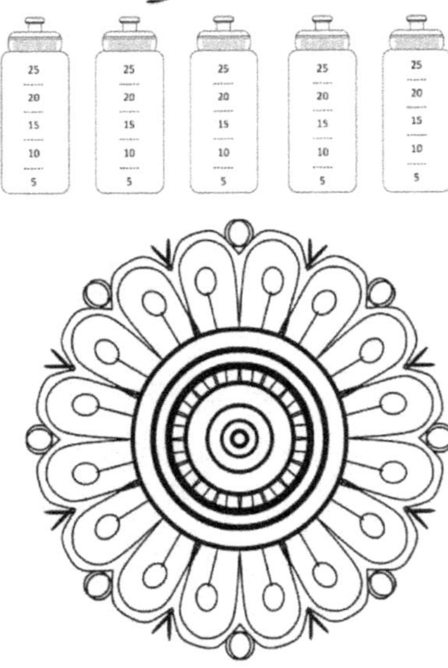

Use this page to record your water intake. Color the bottles as you complete each one. Also each hydration page has a mandala graphic to color. Coloring is a form of meditation. Choose to color this instead of reaching for something to snack on that's not you're your meal plan.

R.O.S.E.S GOAL

Rationale – why are you participating in this 40 day challenge?

____

____

Objective – what do you look to accomplish during the 40 days? What is the end game, goal?

____

____

Strategy – how will you go about completing your objective? What actions will you take.

____

____

Evaluation – how and when will you evaluate you progress? Will you use inches, weight, look, or clothes?

____

____

Schedule – create a schedule for the next 40 days. Include anything that will get in the way of your goal and find a work around.

____

____

Measurements

DATE: __________

Weight: ______

Neck ______

Shoulders ______

Chest ______

Bicep / upper arm left _______ right ______

Forearm left _______ right ______

Waist ______

Hips ______

Thighs left _______ right ______

Calf left _______ right ______

Only I Can Change My Life,
No One Can Do It For Me

Day One ______

5:00 ______
6:00 ______
7:00 ______
8:00 ______
9:00 ______
10:00 ______
11:00 ______
Noon ______
1:00 ______
2:00 ______
3:00 ______
4:00 ______
5:00 ______
6:00 ______
7:00 ______
8:00 ______
9:00 ______
10:00 ______
11:00 ______
Midnight ______

top priorities for today

______
______
______
______
______

Today's victories

What BOLD statement did you make today?

______
______
______
______
______
______
______
______

The Stella Society Training

Exercise	Set 1	Set 2	Set 3	Set 4	Set 5	notes

Time started: ____________ Time ended: ______________

Location: ____

Feelings before training:

Feelings after training

NUTRITION

Meal 1

time eaten: _________

Meal 2

time eaten: _________

Meal 3

time eaten: _________

Meal 4

time eaten: _________

Meal 5

time eaten: _________

Hydration

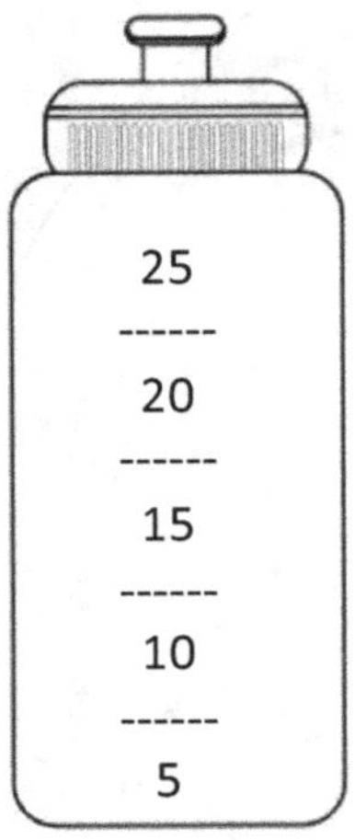

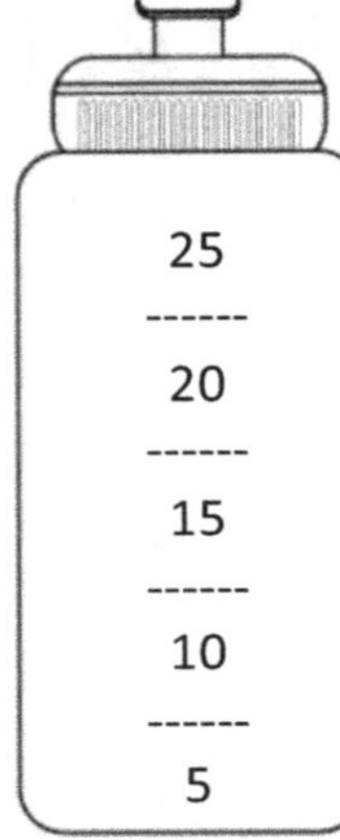

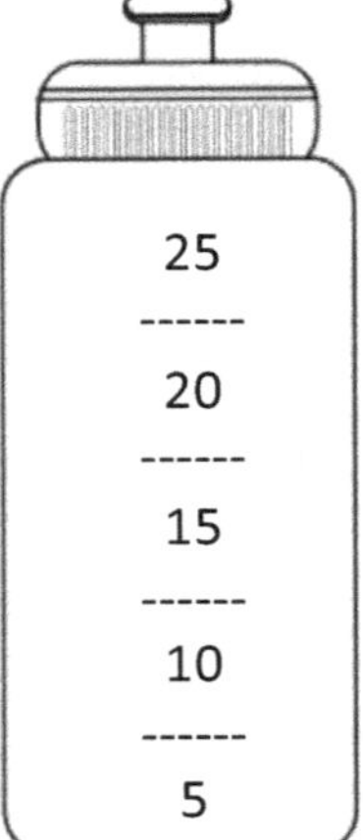

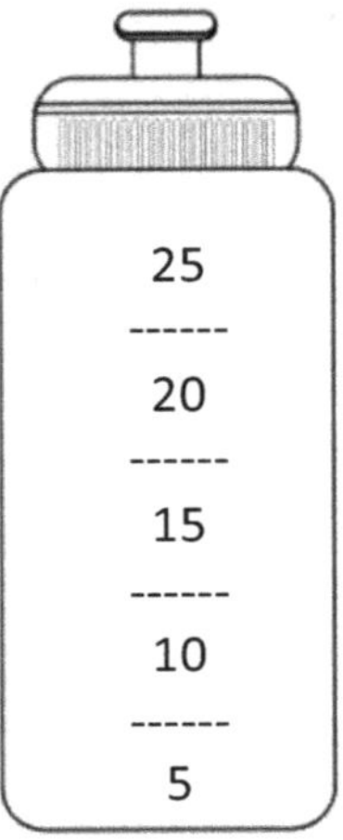

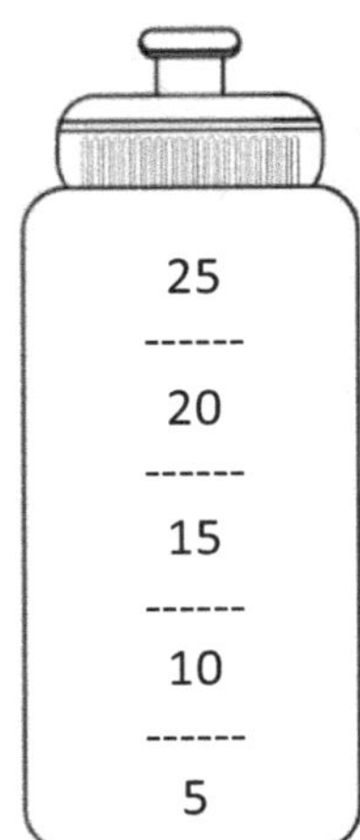

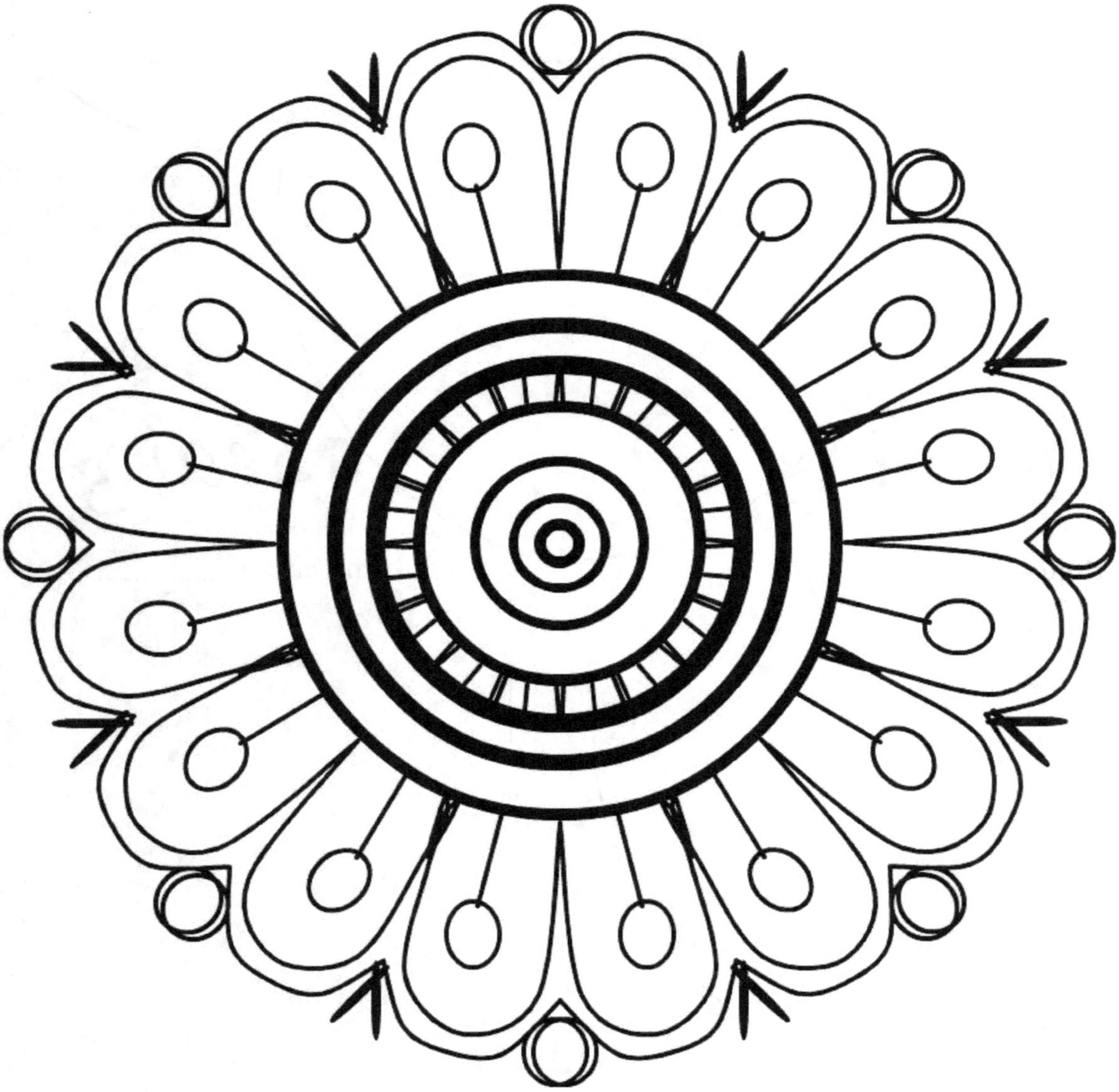

Day Two ______

5:00	______
6:00	______
7:00	______
8:00	______
9:00	______
10:00	______
11:00	______
Noon	______
1:00	______
2:00	______
3:00	______
4:00	______
5:00	______
6:00	______
7:00	______
8:00	______
9:00	______
10:00	______
11:00	______
Midnight	______

top priorities for today

______

______

______

______

Today's victories 

What is one thing that makes you unique??

______

______

______

______

______

______

______

The Stella Society Training

Exercise	Set 1	Set 2	Set 3	Set 4	Set 5	notes

Time started: ____________ Time ended: ______________

Location: ____

Feelings before training: 🙂 😑 ☹️ 😝 😠 😕 😇 😎

Feelings after training 🙂 😑 ☹️ 😝 😠 😕 😇 😎

NUTRITION

Meal 1

time eaten: _________

Meal 2

time eaten: _________

Meal 3

time eaten: _________

Meal 4

time eaten: _________

Meal 5

time eaten: _________

Hydration

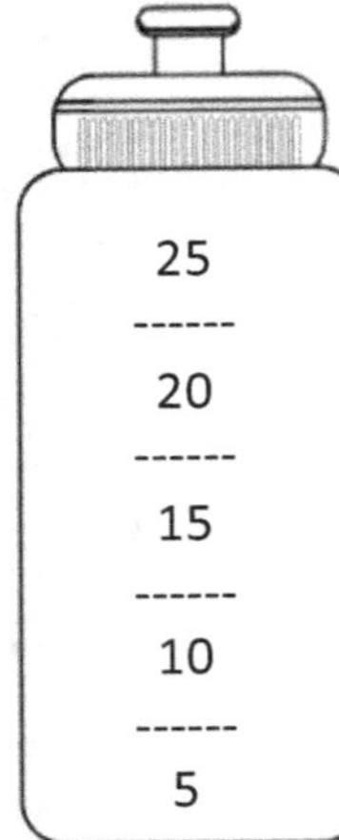

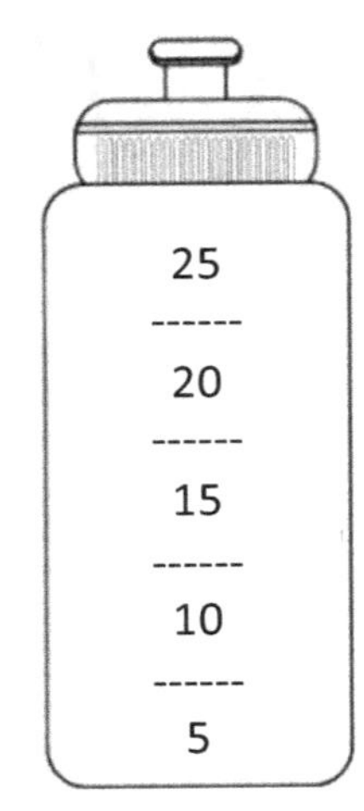

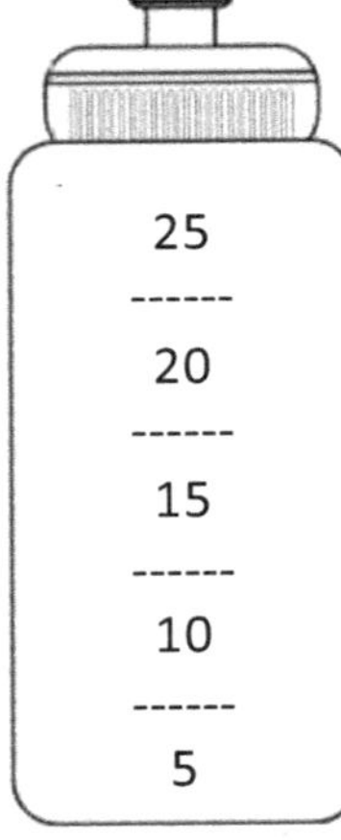

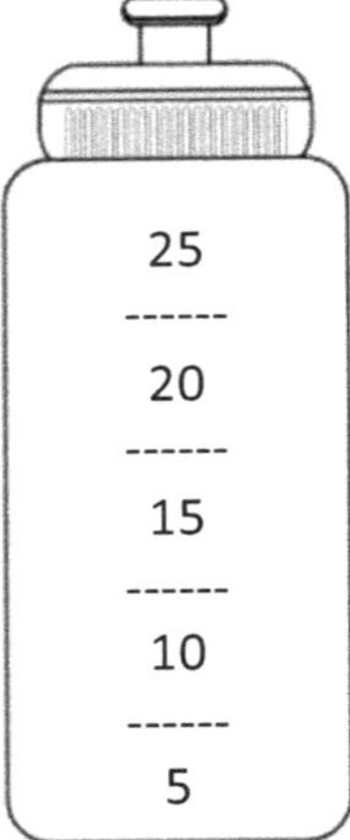

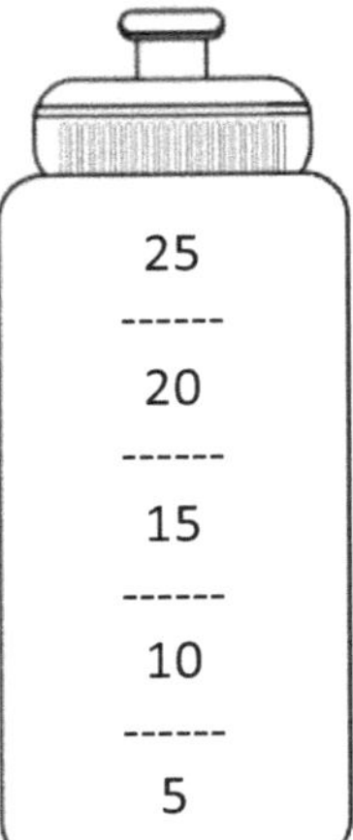

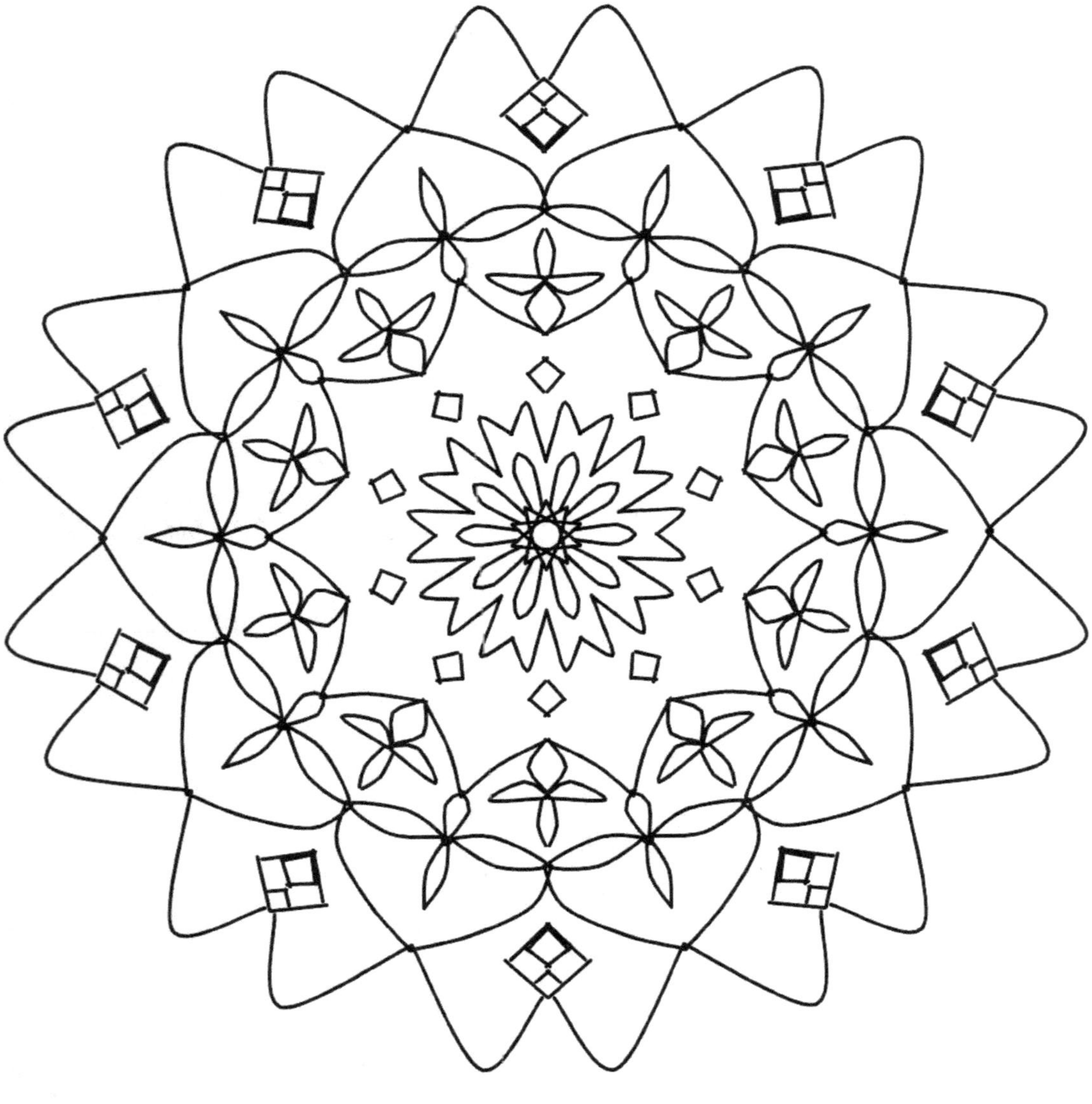

Day Three ______

5:00 ______
6:00 ______
7:00 ______
8:00 ______
9:00 ______
10:00 ______
11:00 ______
Noon ______
1:00 ______
2:00 ______
3:00 ______
4:00 ______
5:00 ______
6:00 ______
7:00 ______
8:00 ______
9:00 ______
10:00 ______
11:00 ______
Midnight ______

top priorities for today

Today's victories

What makes you brave?

The Stella Society Training

Exercise	Set 1	Set 2	Set 3	Set 4	Set 5	notes

Time started: ____________ Time ended: _____________

Location: ____

Feelings before training: ☺ 😑 ☹ 😝 😠 😕 😇 😎

Feelings after training ☺ 😑 ☹ 😝 😠 😕 😇 😎

NUTRITION

Meal 1

time eaten: _________

Meal 2

time eaten: _________

Meal 3

time eaten: _________

Meal 4

time eaten: _________

Meal 5

time eaten: _________

Hydration

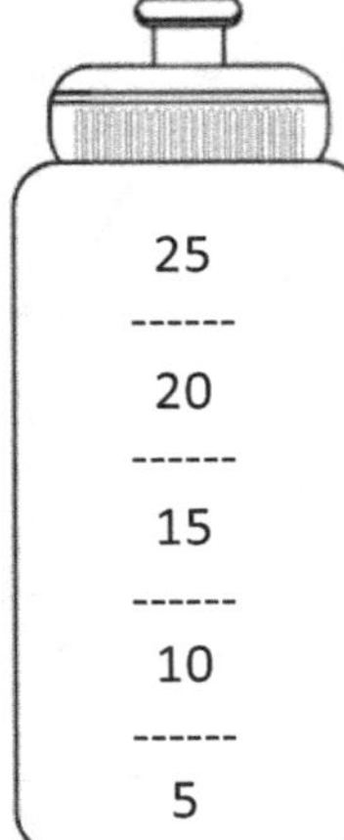

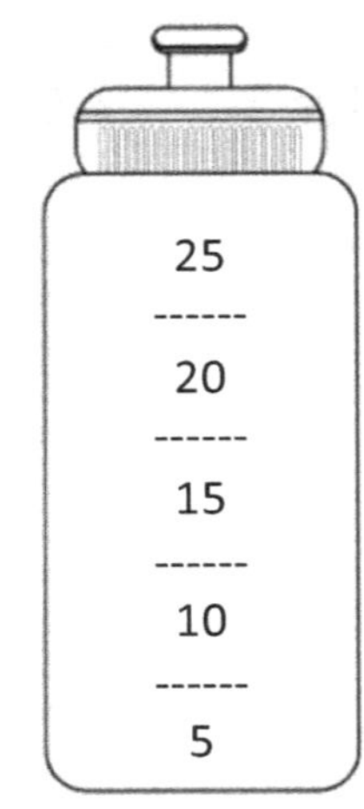

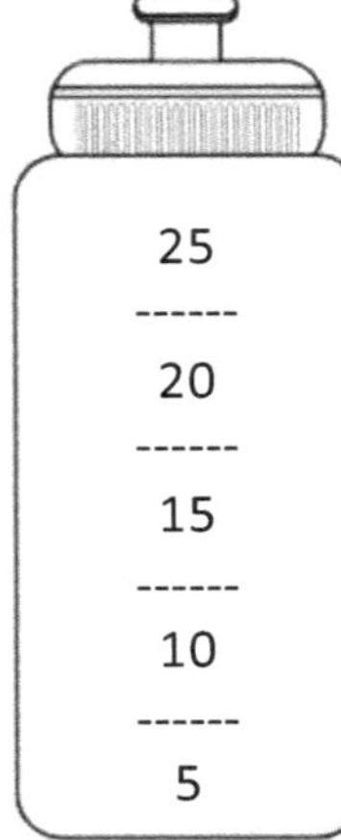

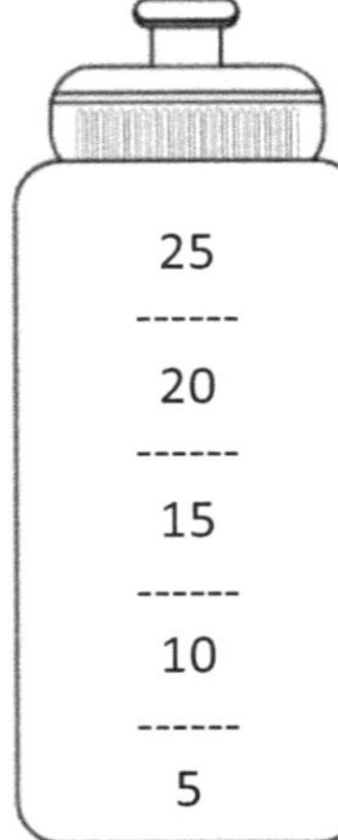

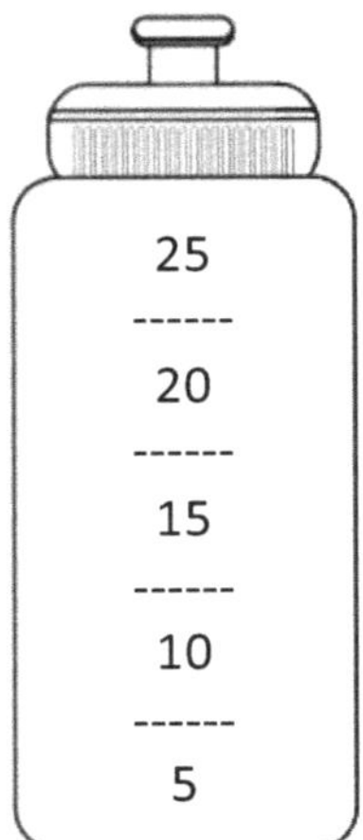

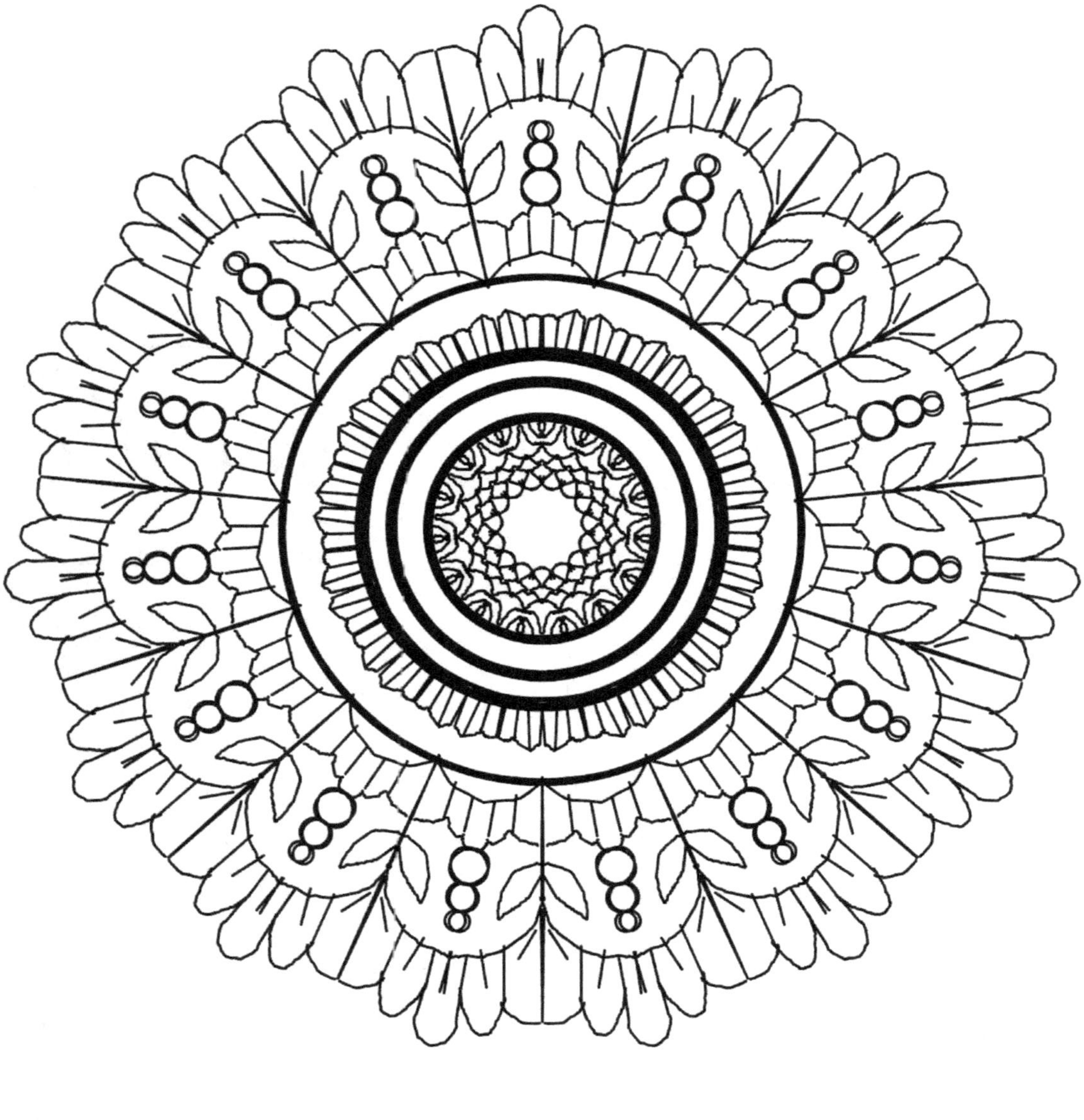

Day Four ______

5:00 ____________________
6:00 ____________________
7:00 ____________________
8:00 ____________________
9:00 ____________________
10:00 ____________________
11:00 ____________________
Noon ____________________
1:00 ____________________
2:00 ____________________
3:00 ____________________
4:00 ____________________
5:00 ____________________
6:00 ____________________
7:00 ____________________
8:00 ____________________
9:00 ____________________
10:00 ____________________
11:00 ____________________
Midnight ____________________

top priorities for today

Today's victories

What did you commit to today that will make for a better tomorrow?

The Stella Society Training

Exercise	Set 1	Set 2	Set 3	Set 4	Set 5	notes

Time started: ____________ Time ended: _____________

Location: ____

Feelings before training: 😊 😑 ☹️ 😝 😠 😕 😇 😎

Feelings aftertraining 😊 😑 ☹️ 😝 😠 😕 😇 😎

NUTRITION

Meal 1

time eaten: _________

Meal 2

time eaten: _________

Meal 3

time eaten: _________

Meal 4

time eaten: _________

Meal 5

time eaten: _________

Hydration

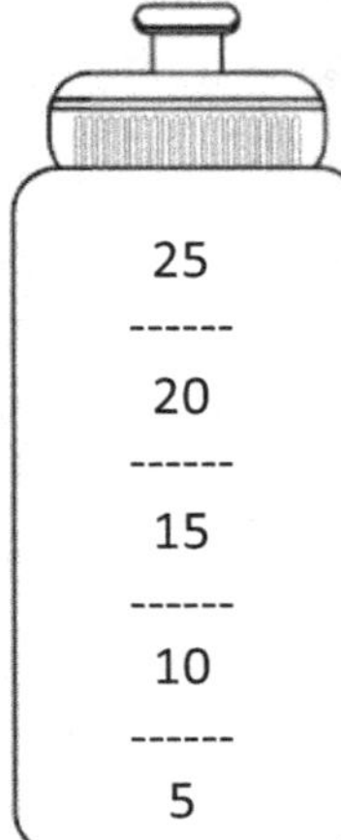

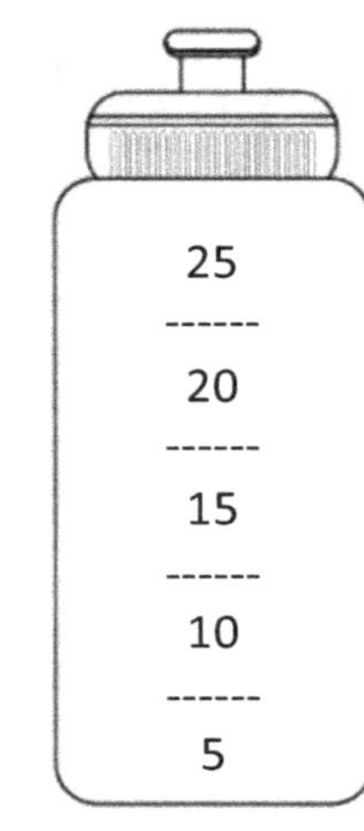

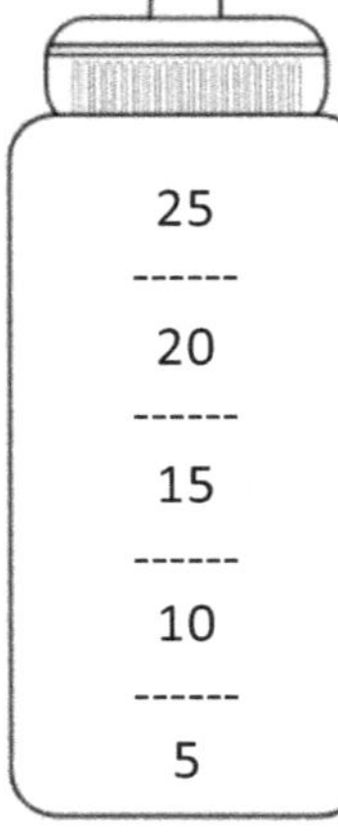

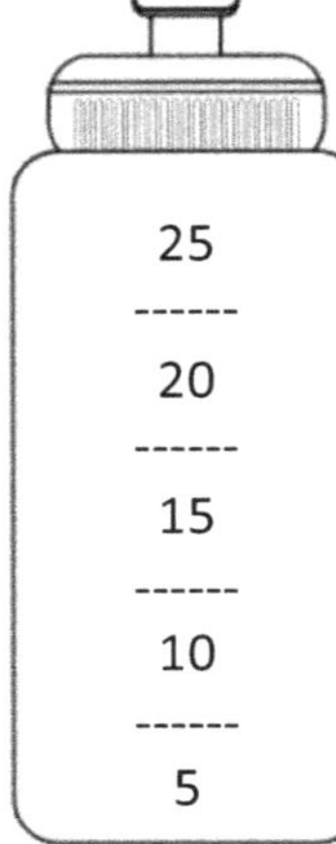

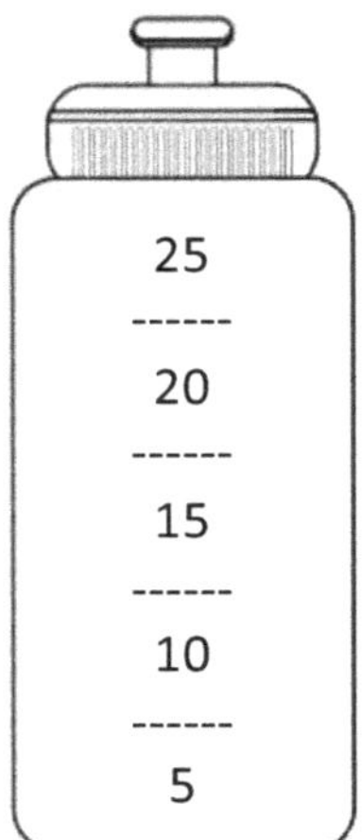

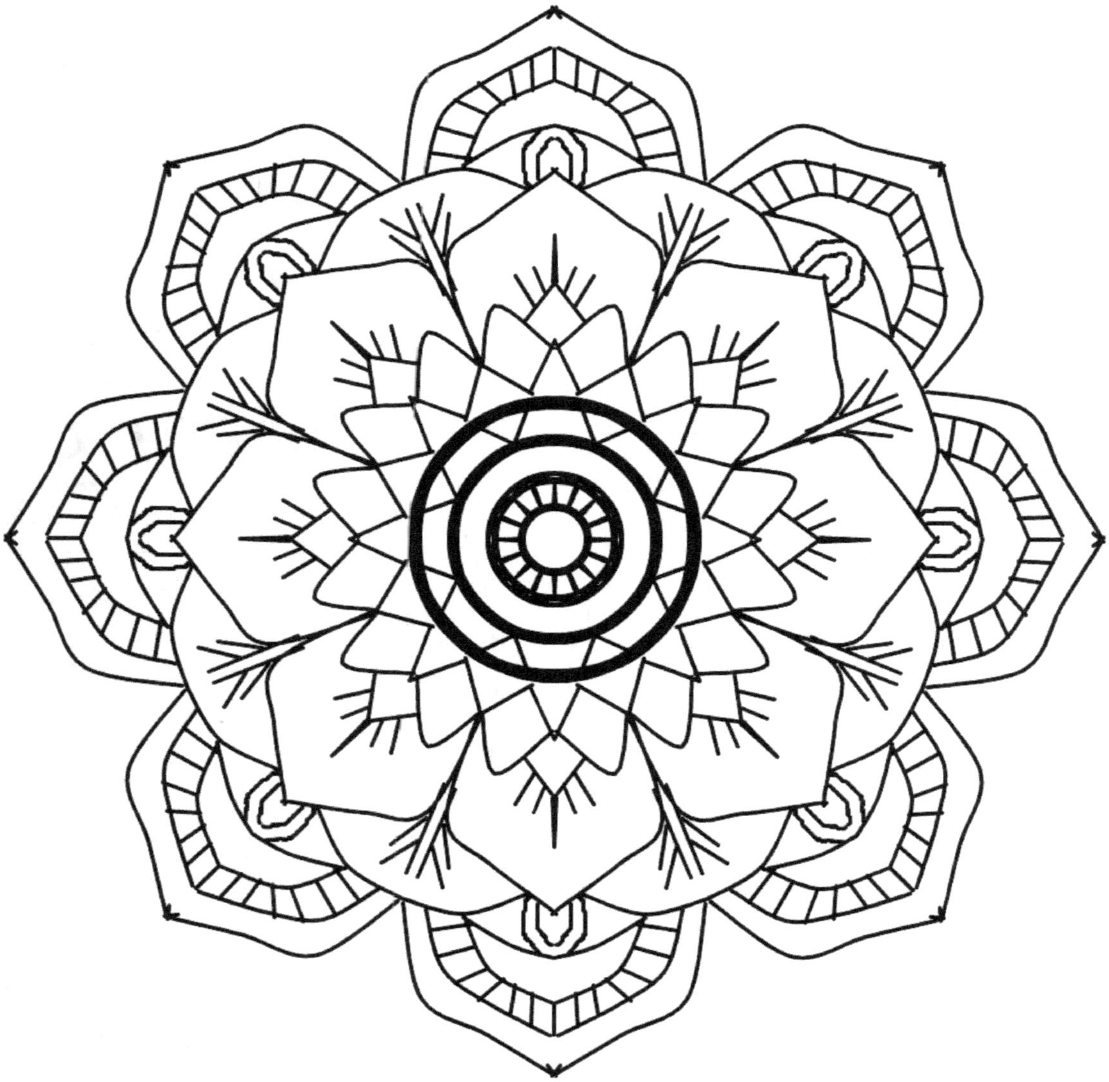

Day Five ______

5:00 ______

6:00 ______

7:00 ______

8:00 ______

9:00 ______

10:00 ______

11:00 ______

Noon ______

1:00 ______

2:00 ______

3:00 ______

4:00 ______

5:00 ______

6:00 ______

7:00 ______

8:00 ______

9:00 ______

10:00 ______

11:00 ______

Midnight ______

top priorities for today

______

______

______

______

Today's victories

Who is the wisest person you know?
Talk to them today.

______

______

______

______

______

______

______

The Stella Society Training

Exercise	Set 1	Set 2	Set 3	Set 4	Set 5	notes

Time started: ____________ Time ended: ______________

Location: ____

Feelings before training:

Feelings after training

NUTRITION

Meal 1

time eaten: _________

Meal 2

time eaten: _________

Meal 3

time eaten: _________

Meal 4

time eaten: _________

Meal 5

time eaten: _________

Hydration

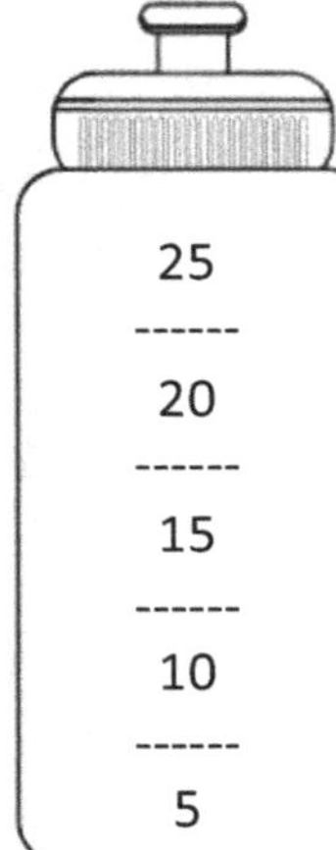

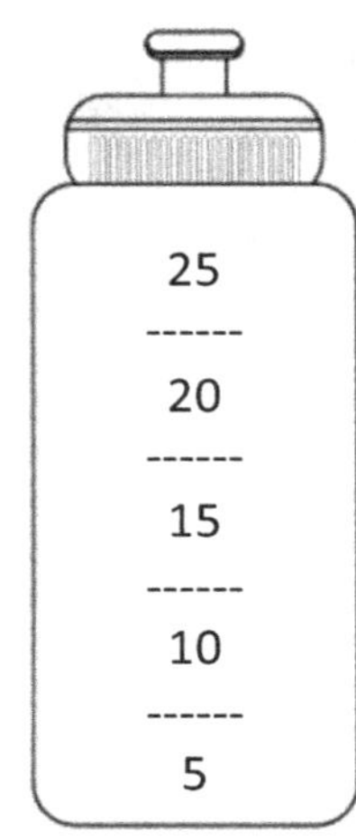

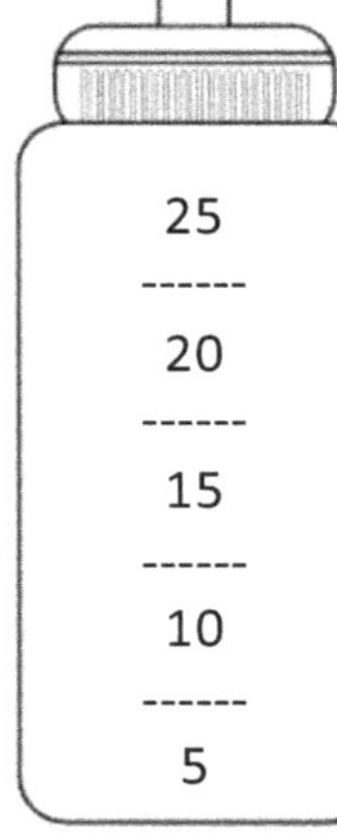

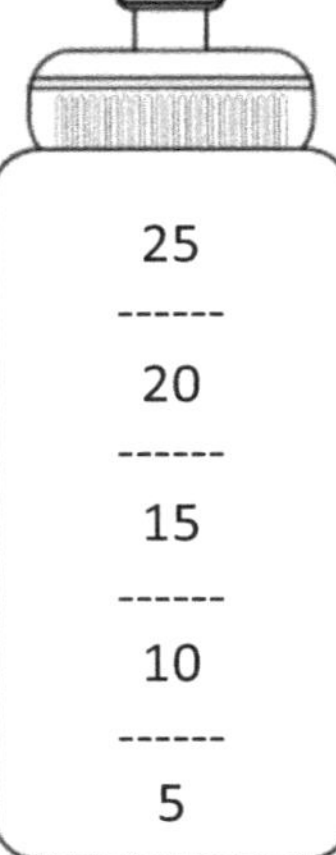

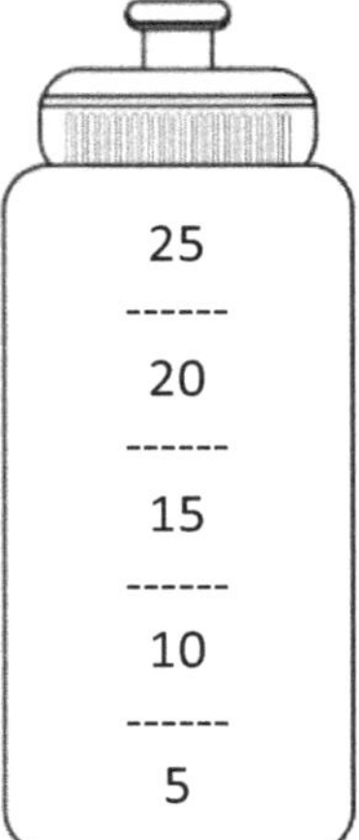

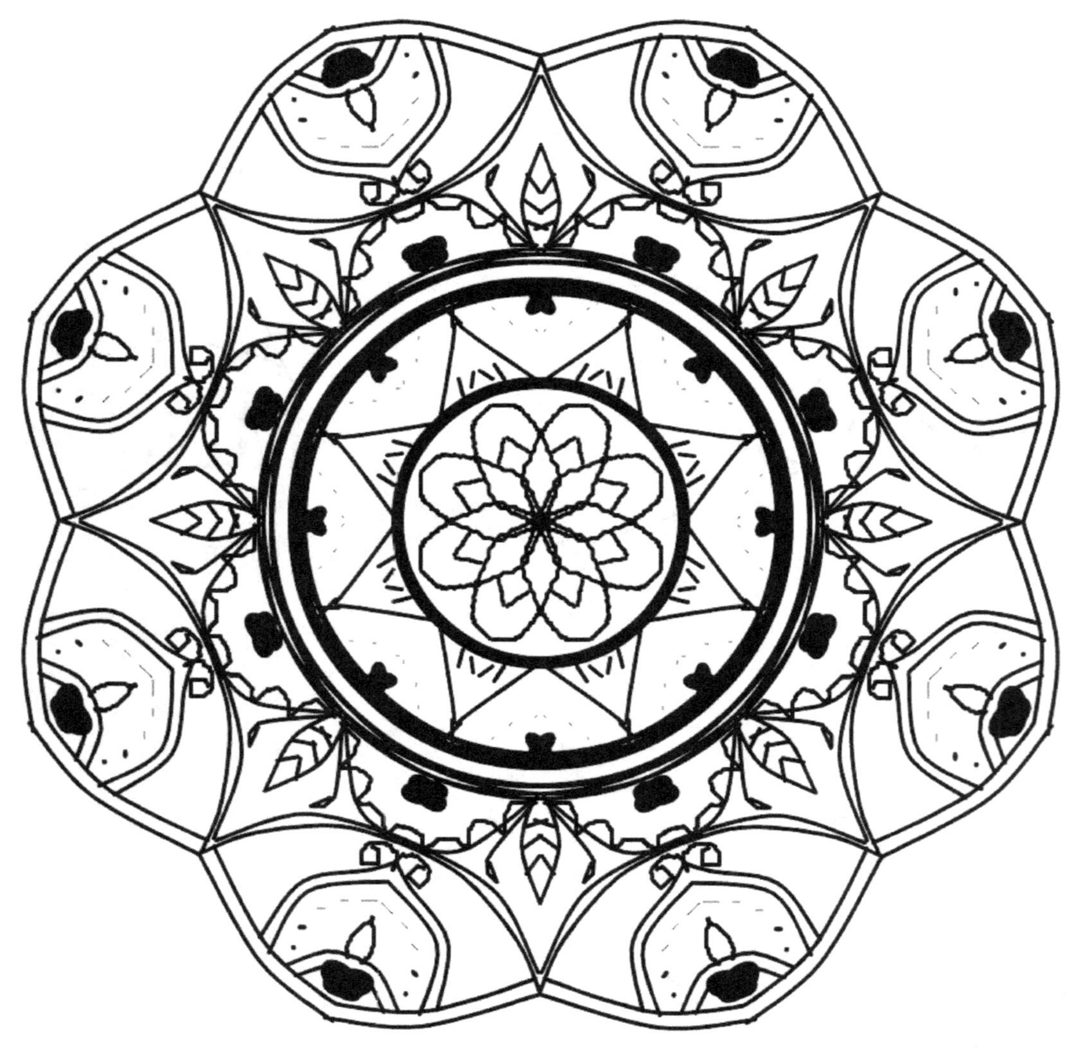

Day Six ______

5:00 ______

6:00 ______

7:00 ______

8:00 ______

9:00 ______

10:00 ______

11:00 ______

Noon ______

1:00 ______

2:00 ______

3:00 ______

4:00 ______

5:00 ______

6:00 ______

7:00 ______

8:00 ______

9:00 ______

10:00 ______

11:00 ______

Midnight ______

top priorities for today

______

______

______

______

______

Today's victories

What is your biggest fear and how do you get over it?

______

______

______

______

______

______

______

______

BE FEARLESS

The Stella Society Training

Exercise	Set 1	Set 2	Set 3	Set 4	Set 5	notes

Time started: ____________ Time ended: _____________

Location: ____

Feelings before training: ☺ 😑 ☹ 😝 😠 😕 😇 😎

Feelings after training ☺ 😑 ☹ 😝 😠 😕 😇 😎

NUTRITION

Meal 1

time eaten: _________

Meal 2

time eaten: _________

Meal 3

time eaten: _________

Meal 4

time eaten: _________

Meal 5

time eaten: _________

Hydration

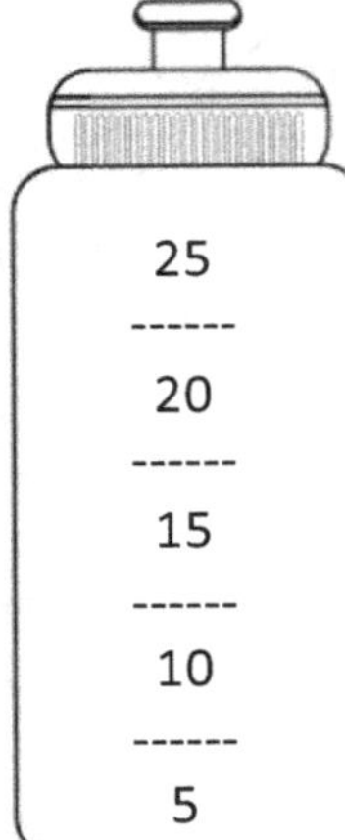

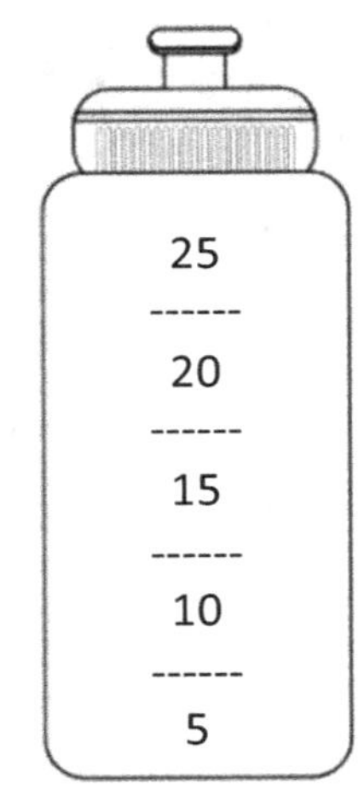

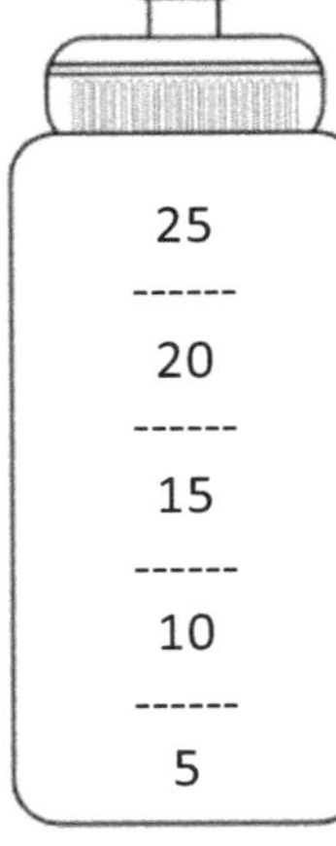

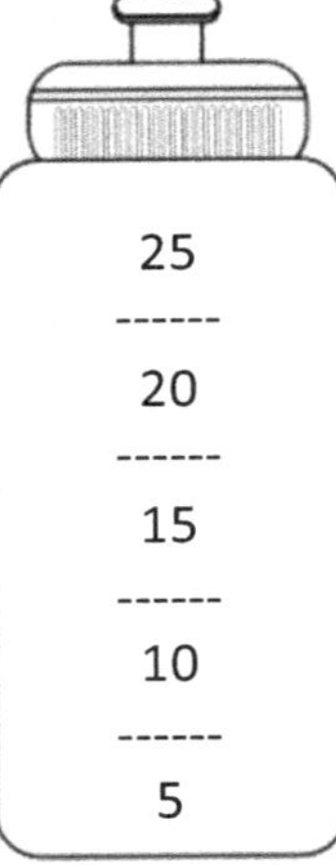

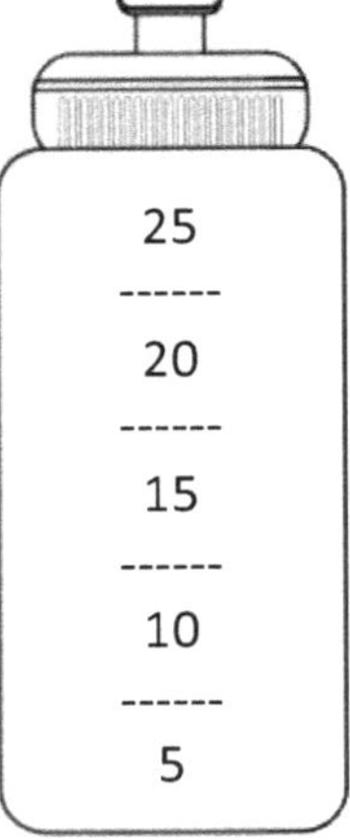

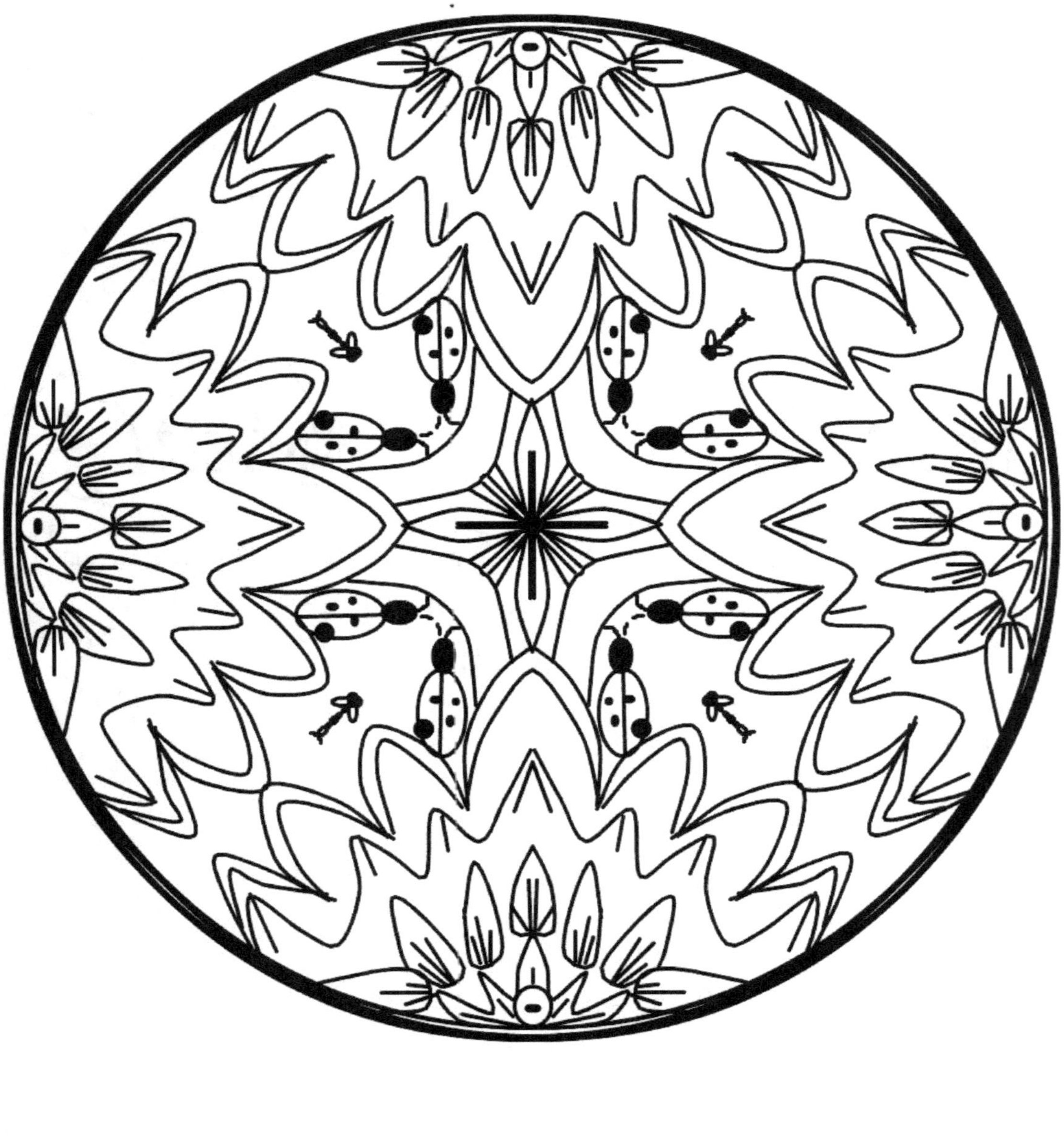

Day Seven ______

5:00 ______
6:00 ______
7:00 ______
8:00 ______
9:00 ______
10:00 ______
11:00 ______
Noon ______
1:00 ______
2:00 ______
3:00 ______
4:00 ______
5:00 ______
6:00 ______
7:00 ______
8:00 ______
9:00 ______
10:00 ______
11:00 ______
Midnight ______

top priorities for today

______
______
______
______
______

Today's victories

Where does your strength come from?

______
______
______
______
______
______
______
______

BE STRONG

The Stella Society Training

Exercise	Set 1	Set 2	Set 3	Set 4	Set 5	notes

Time started: ____________ Time ended: ______________

Location: ____

Feelings before training: 😊 😐 ☹️ 😝 😠 😕 😇 😎

Feelings after training 😊 😐 ☹️ 😝 😠 😕 😇 😎

NUTRITION

Meal 1

time eaten: _________

Meal 2

time eaten: _________

Meal 3

time eaten: _________

Meal 4

time eaten: _________

Meal 5

time eaten: _________

Hydration

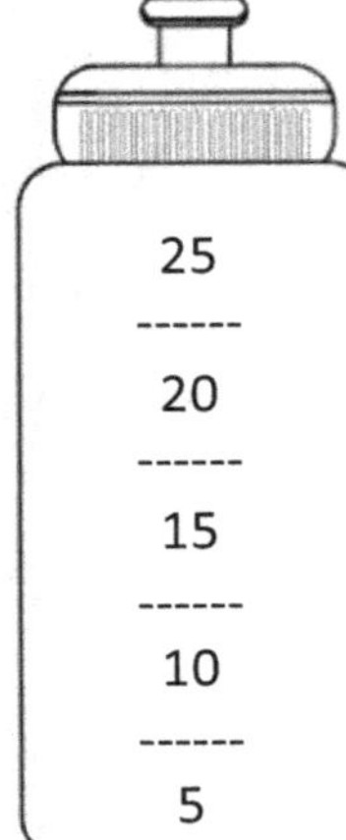

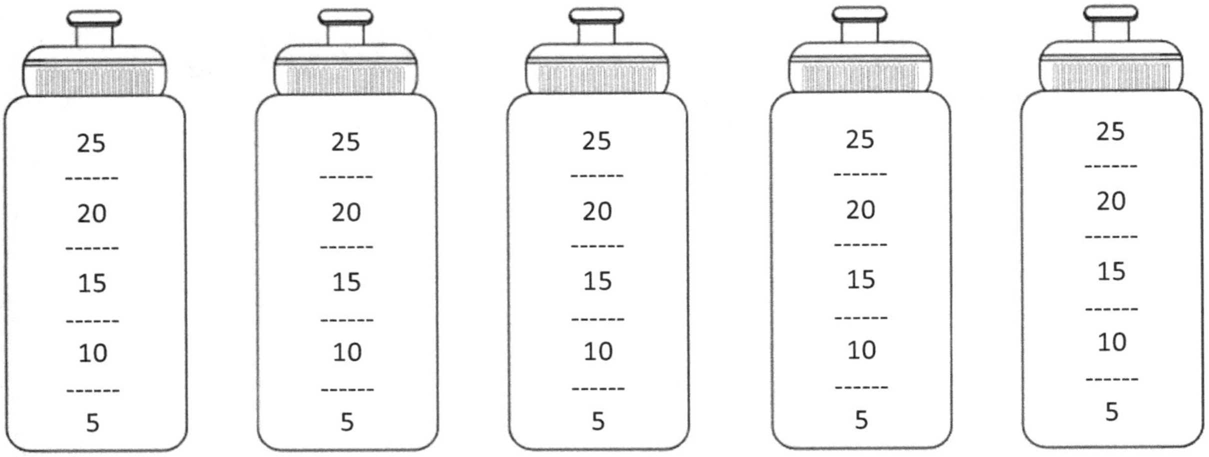

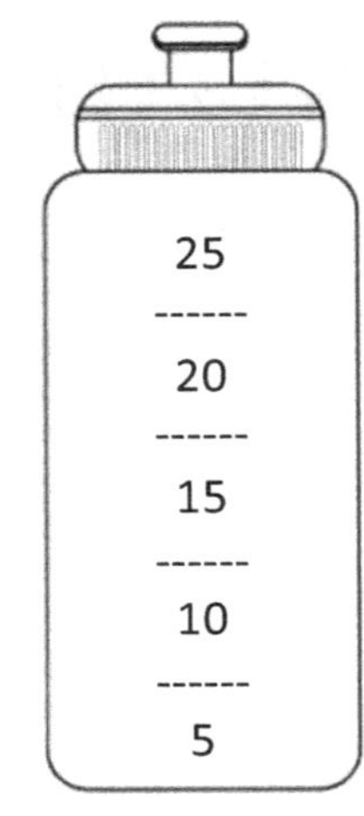

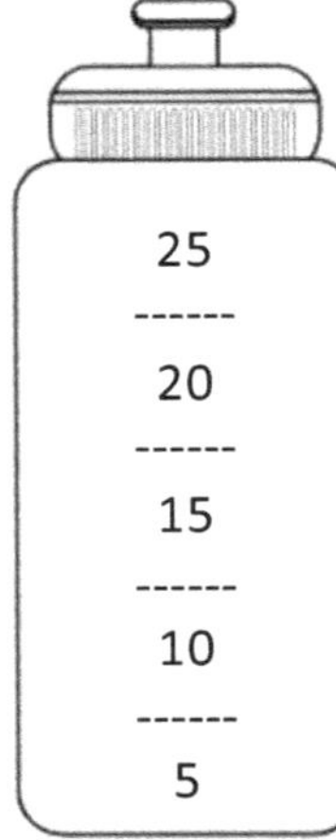

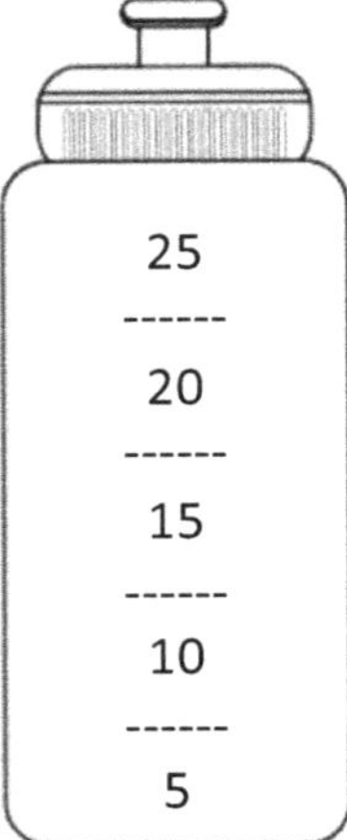

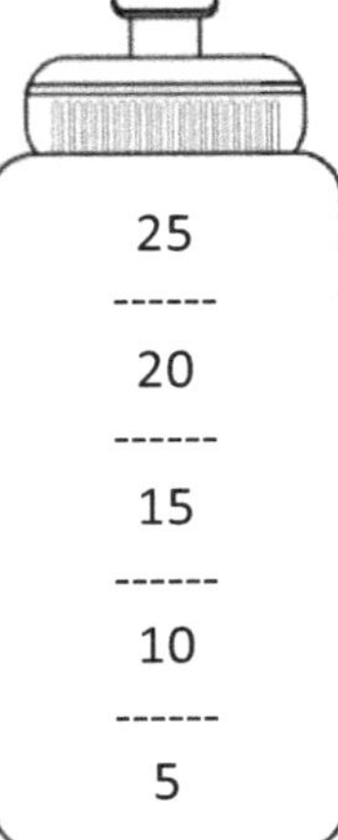

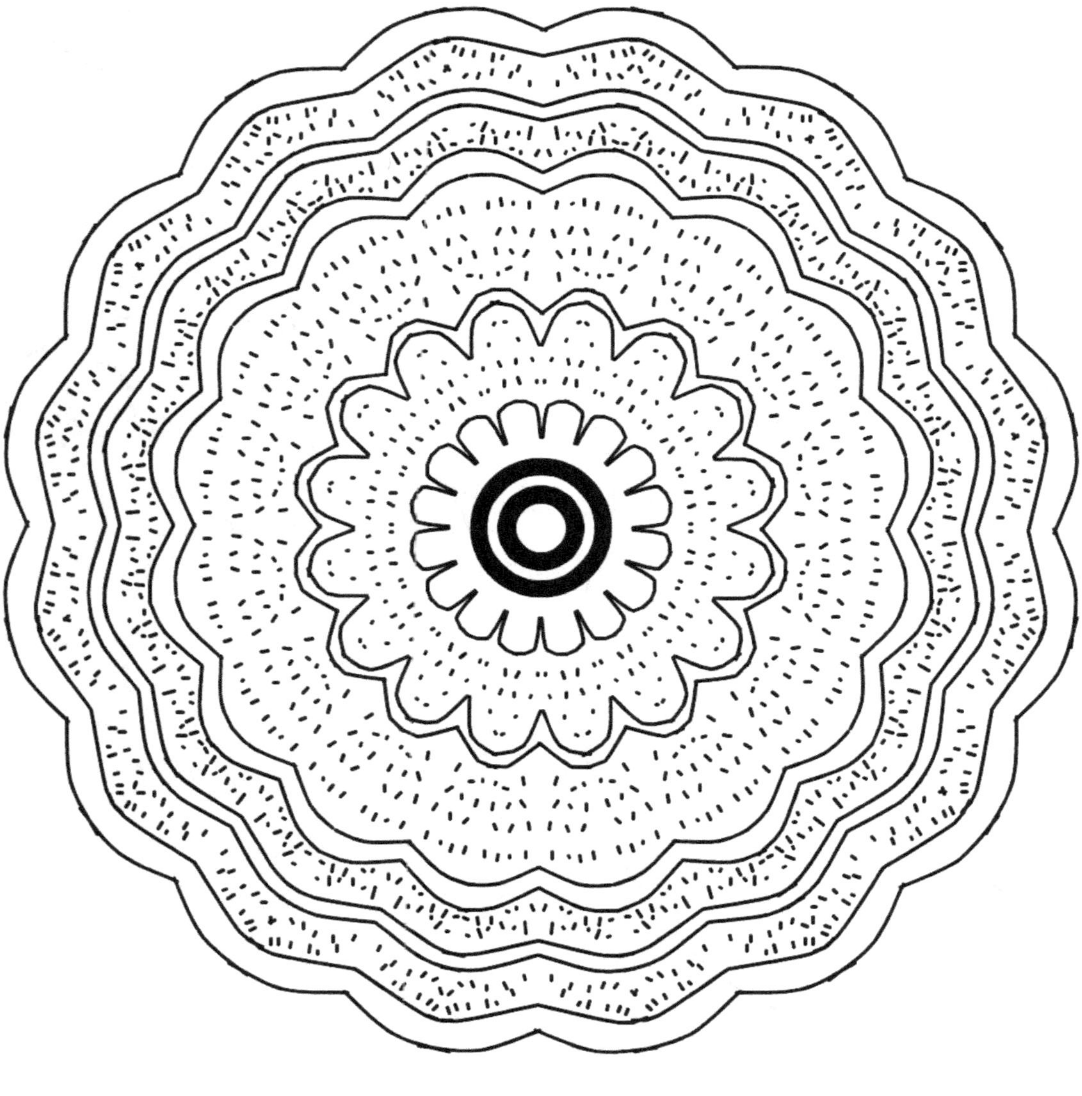

Day Eight ______

5:00 ____________________

6:00 ____________________

7:00 ____________________

8:00 ____________________

9:00 ____________________

10:00 ____________________

11:00 ____________________

Noon ____________________

1:00 ____________________

2:00 ____________________

3:00 ____________________

4:00 ____________________

5:00 ____________________

6:00 ____________________

7:00 ____________________

8:00 ____________________

9:00 ____________________

10:00 ____________________

11:00 ____________________

Midnight ____________________

top priorities for today

____

____

____

____

____

Today's victories

What motivates you to be the best version of you?

____

____

____

____

____

____

____

____

The Stella Society Training

Exercise	Set 1	Set 2	Set 3	Set 4	Set 5	notes

Time started: ____________ Time ended: _____________

Location: ____

Feelings before training: ☺ 😑 ☹ 😝 😠 😕 😇 😎

Feelings after training ☺ 😑 ☹ 😝 😠 😕 😇 😎

NUTRITION

Meal 1

time eaten: _________

Meal 2

time eaten: _________

Meal 3

time eaten: _________

Meal 4

time eaten: _________

Meal 5

time eaten: _________

Hydration

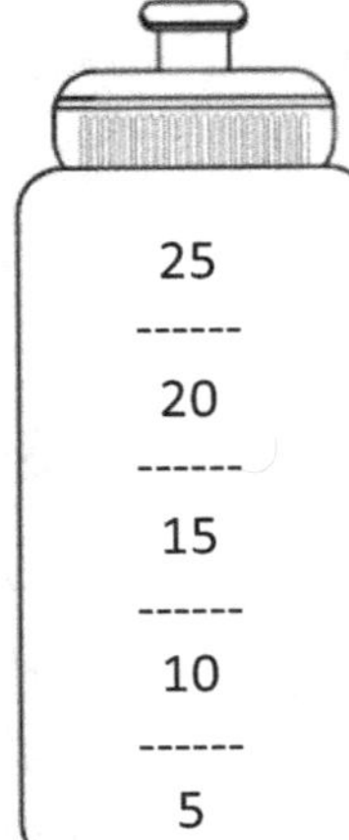

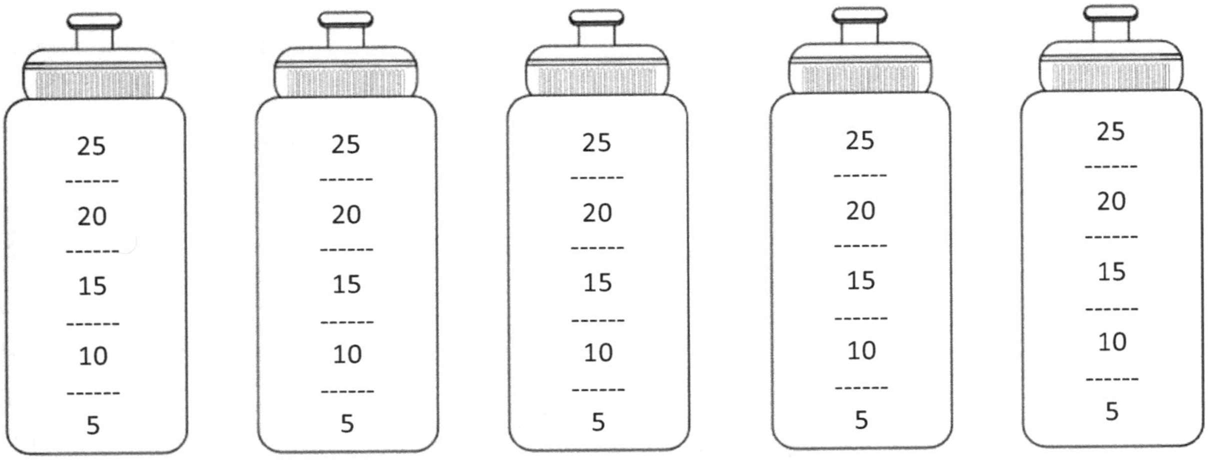

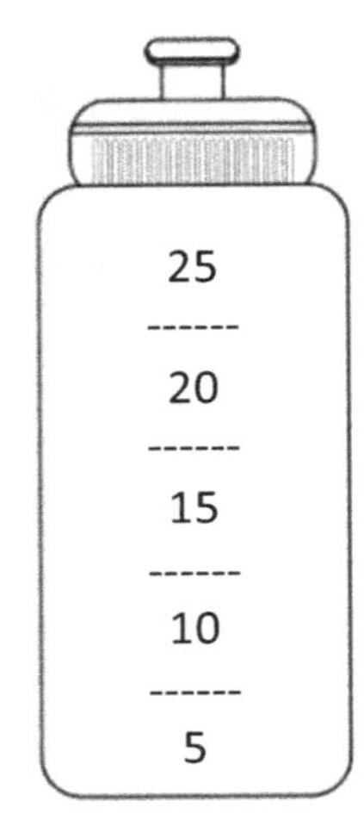

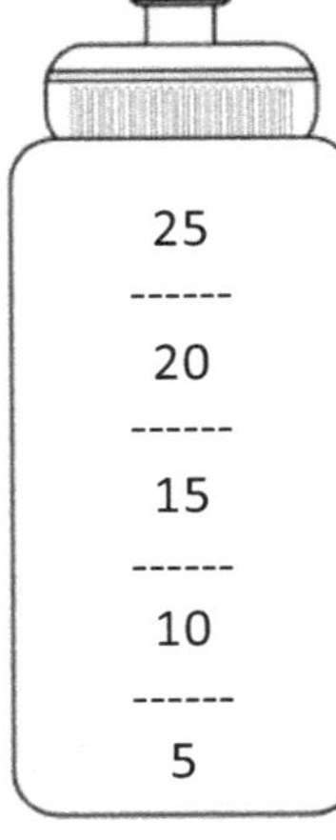

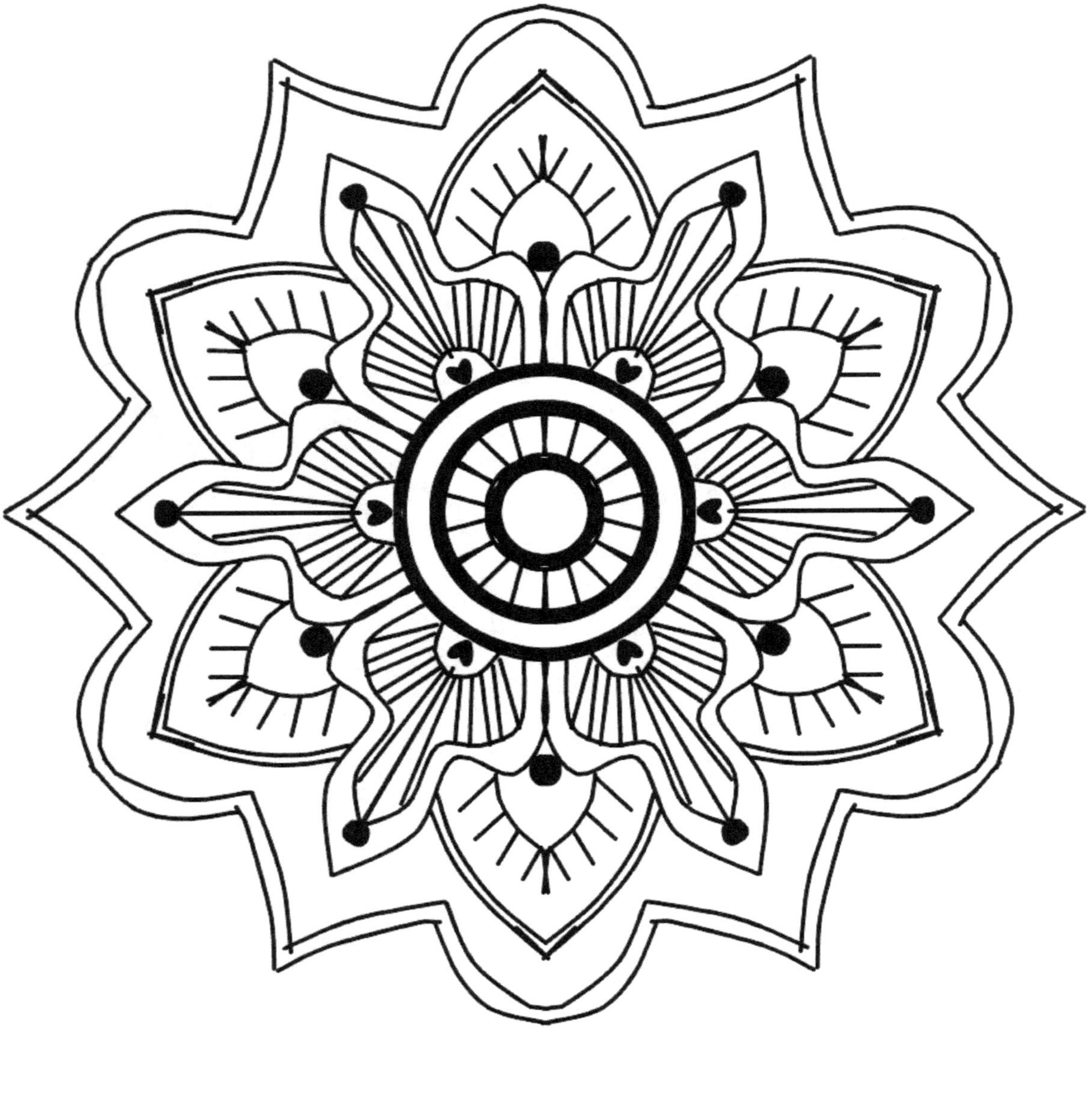

25

20

15

10

5

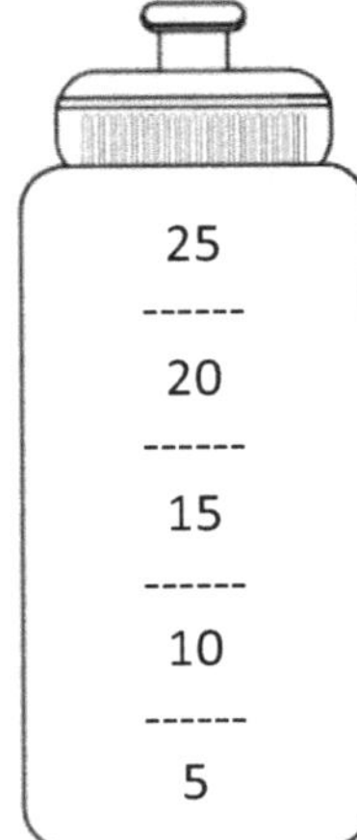

Day Nine ______

5:00 ______
6:00 ______
7:00 ______
8:00 ______
9:00 ______
10:00 ______
11:00 ______
Noon ______
1:00 ______
2:00 ______
3:00 ______
4:00 ______
5:00 ______
6:00 ______
7:00 ______
8:00 ______
9:00 ______
10:00 ______
11:00 ______
Midnight ______

top priorities for today

______
______
______
______
______

Today's victories

How will you be consistent this week?

______
______
______
______
______
______
______
______

The Stella Society Training

Exercise	Set 1	Set 2	Set 3	Set 4	Set 5	notes

Time started: ____________ Time ended: _____________

Location: ____

Feelings before training: ☺ 😑 ☹ 😝 😠 😕 😇 😎

Feelings after training ☺ 😑 ☹ 😝 😠 😕 😇 😎

NUTRITION

Meal 1

time eaten: _________

Meal 2

time eaten: _________

Meal 3

time eaten: _________

Meal 4

time eaten: _________

Meal 5

time eaten: _________

Hydration

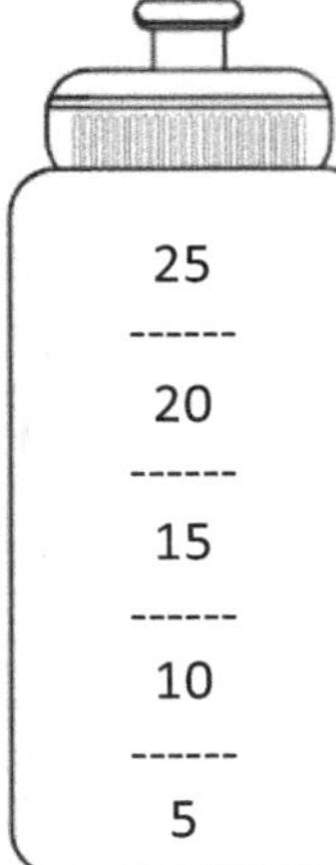

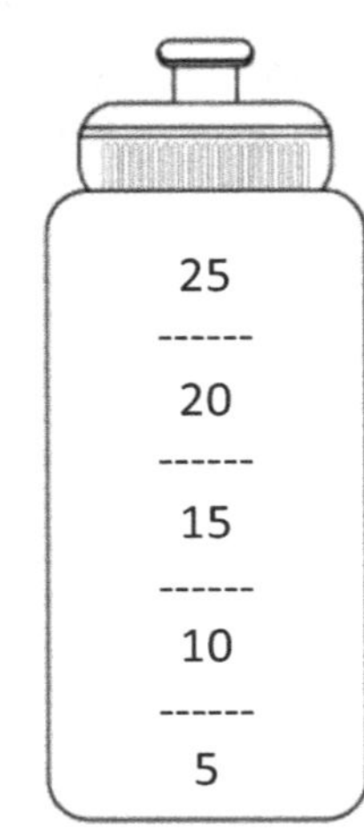

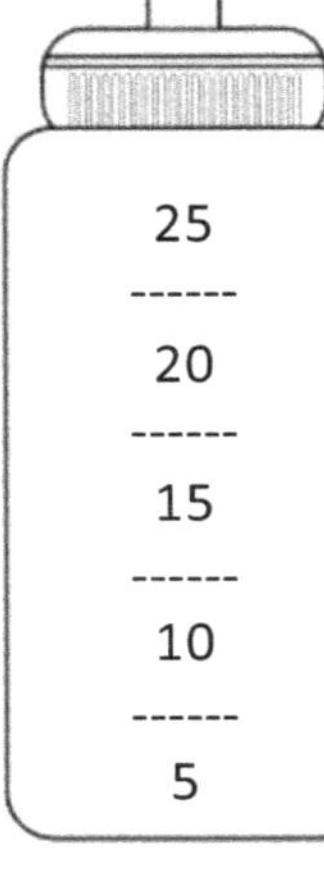

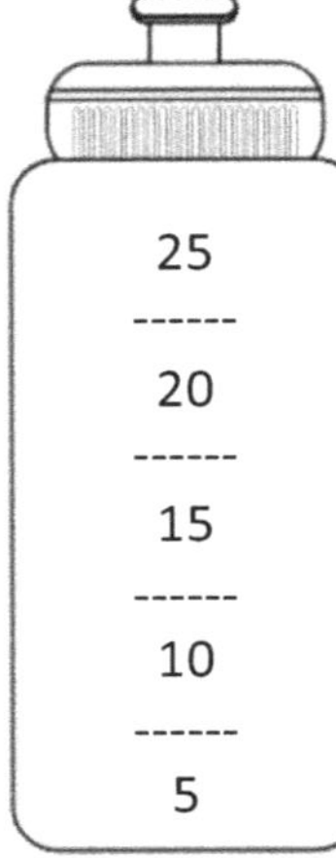

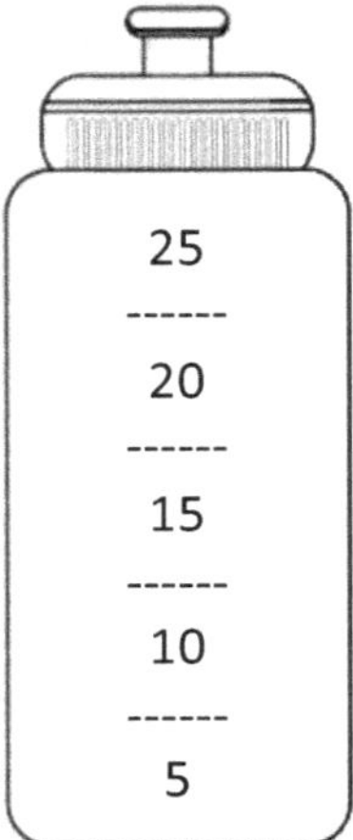

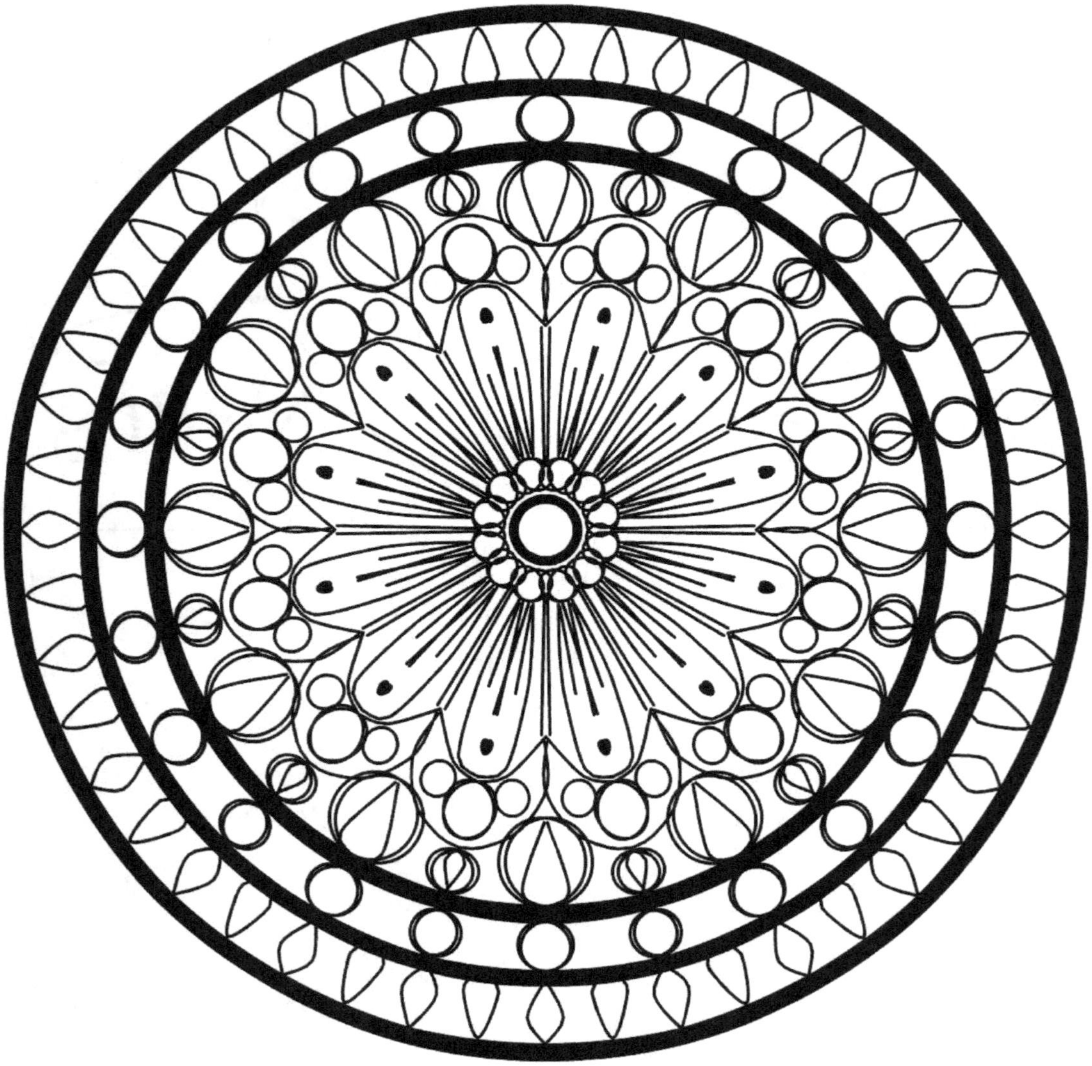

Day Ten ______

5:00 ______
6:00 ______
7:00 ______
8:00 ______
9:00 ______
10:00 ______
11:00 ______
Noon ______
1:00 ______
2:00 ______
3:00 ______
4:00 ______
5:00 ______
6:00 ______
7:00 ______
8:00 ______
9:00 ______
10:00 ______
11:00 ______
Midnight ______

top priorities for today

______
______
______
______
______

Today's victories

List 5 ways you are loving.

______
______
______
______
______
______
______
______

BE LOVING

The Stella Society Training

Exercise	Set 1	Set 2	Set 3	Set 4	Set 5	notes

Time started: ____________ Time ended: _____________

Location: ____

Feelings before training:

Feelings after training

NUTRITION

Meal 1

time eaten: _________

Meal 2

time eaten: _________

Meal 3

time eaten: _________

Meal 4

time eaten: _________

Meal 5

time eaten: _________

Hydration

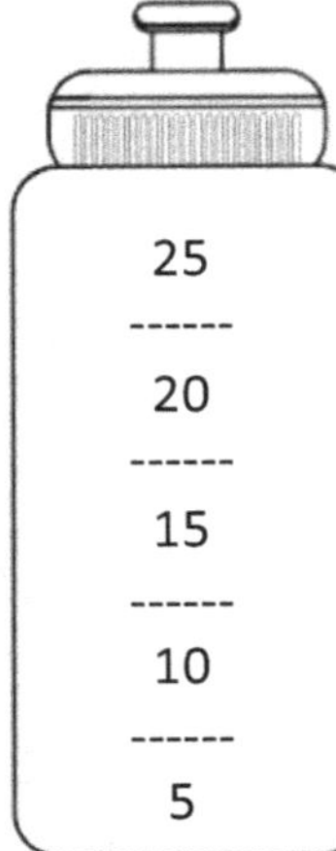

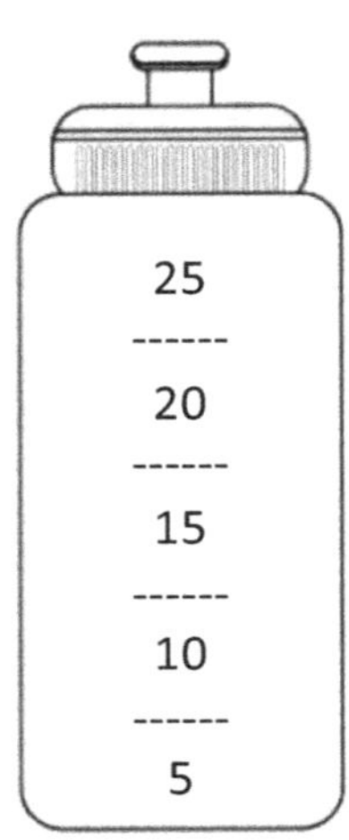

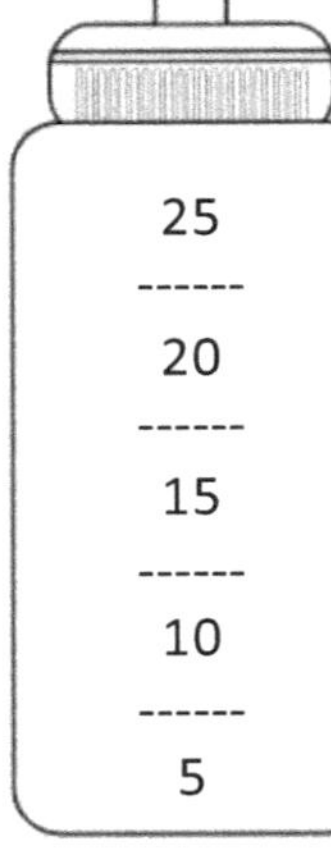

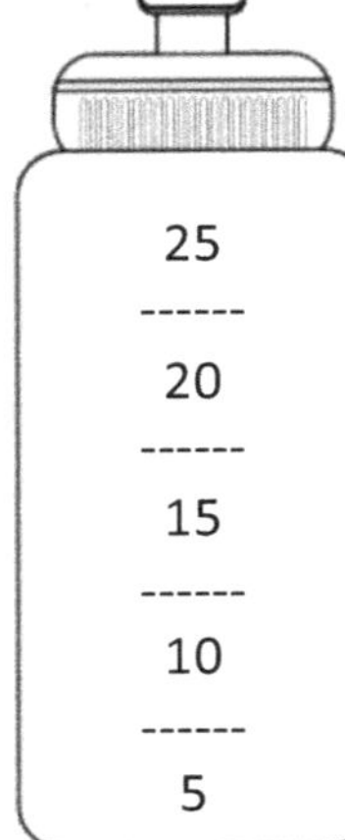

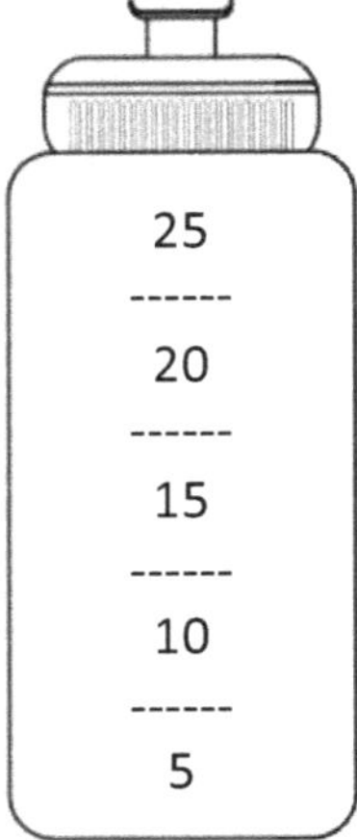

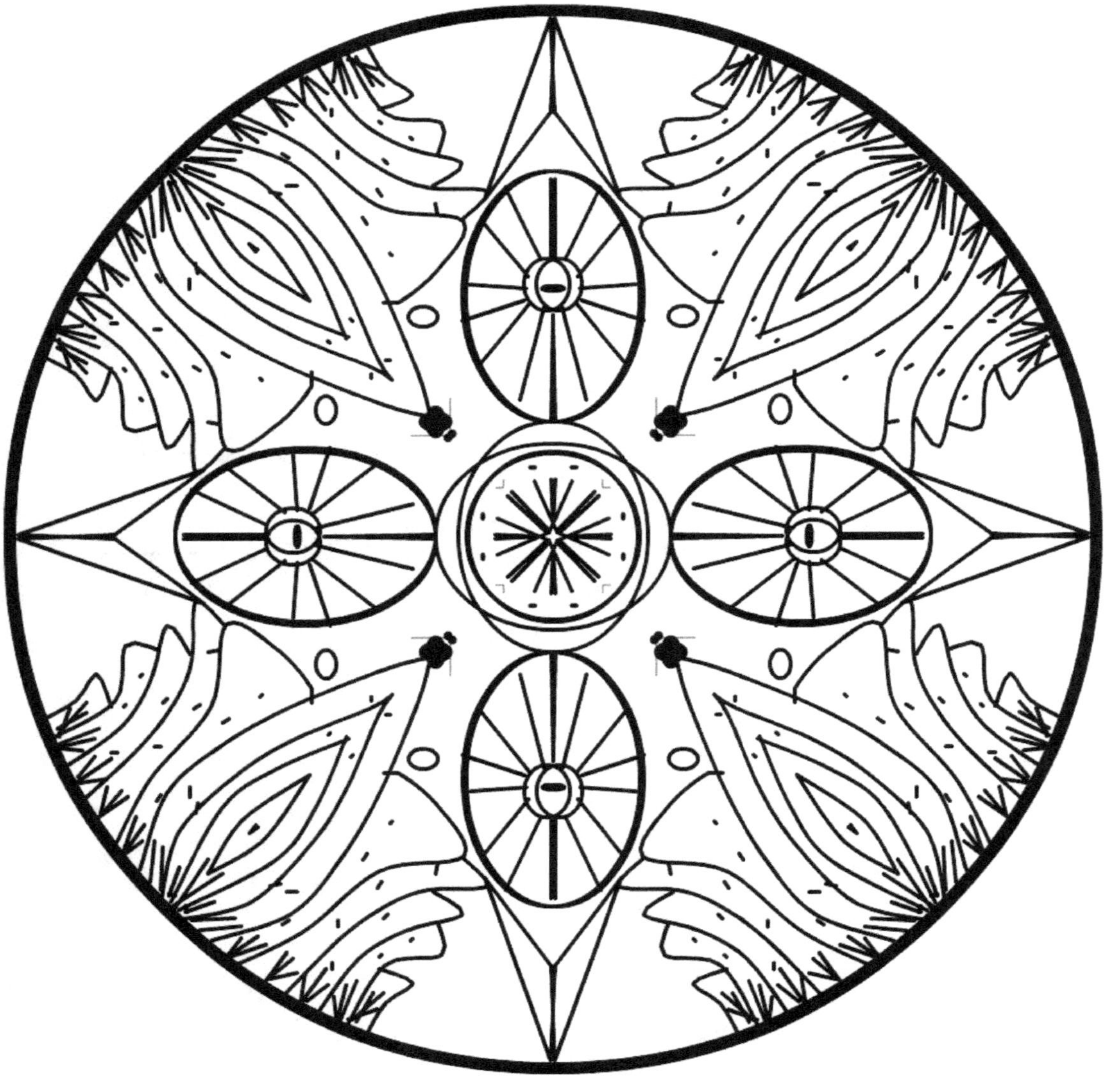

Measurements

PROGRESS CHECK

DATE: ___________

Weight: ______

Neck ______

Shoulders ______

Chest ______

Bicep / upper arm left _______ right ______

Forearm left _______ right ______

Waist ______

Hips ______

Thighs left _______ right ____

Calf left _______ right ______

The Struggle You Are In Today, Is Developing The Strength You Need for Tomorrow.

Day Eleven ______

5:00 ______
6:00 ______
7:00 ______
8:00 ______
9:00 ______
10:00 ______
11:00 ______
Noon ______
1:00 ______
2:00 ______
3:00 ______
4:00 ______
5:00 ______
6:00 ______
7:00 ______
8:00 ______
9:00 ______
10:00 ______
11:00 ______
Midnight ______

top priorities for today

______
______
______
______
______

Today's victories

Give out as many hugs as you can today. How many did you give?

______
______
______
______
______
______
______
______

The Stella Society Training

Exercise	Set 1	Set 2	Set 3	Set 4	Set 5	notes

Time started: ____________ Time ended: ______________

Location: ____

Feelings before training: 🙂 😑 🙁 😝 😠 😕 😇 😎

Feelings after training 🙂 😑 🙁 😝 😠 😕 😇 😎

NUTRITION

Meal 1

time eaten: _________

Meal 2

time eaten: _________

Meal 3

time eaten: _________

Meal 4

time eaten: _________

Meal 5

time eaten: _________

Hydration

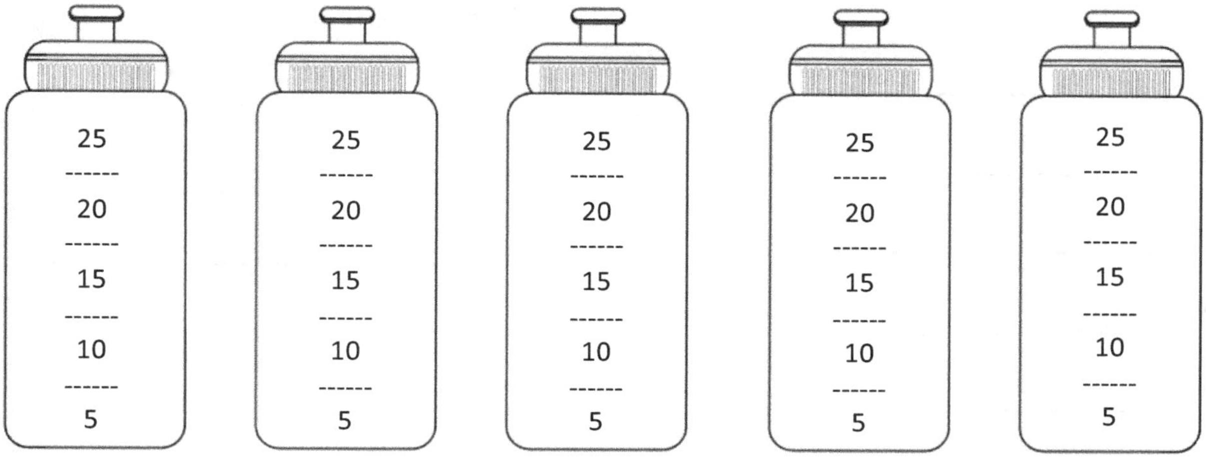

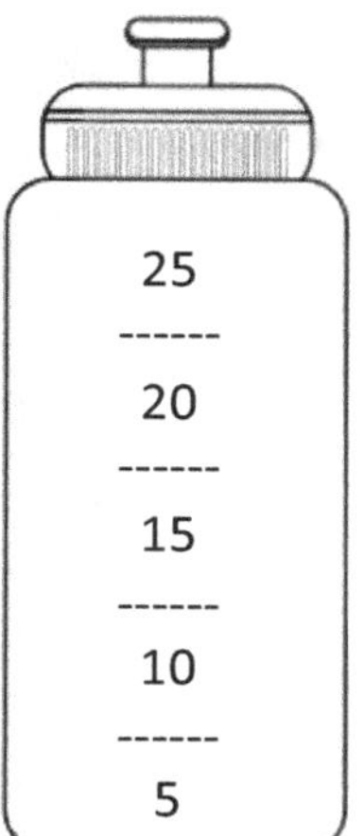

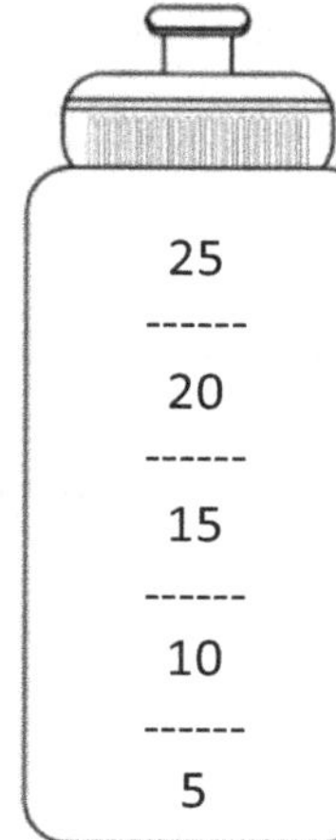

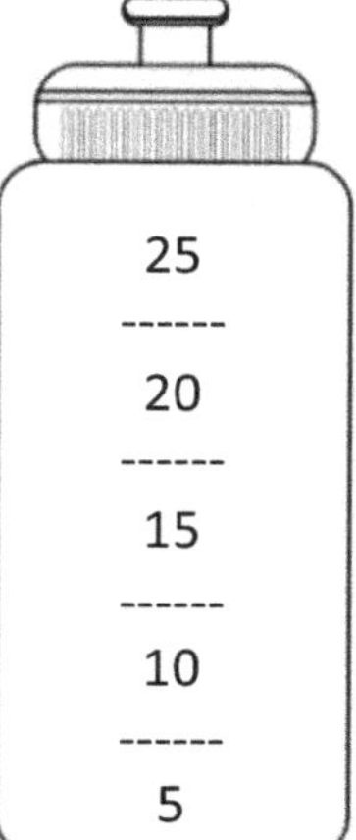

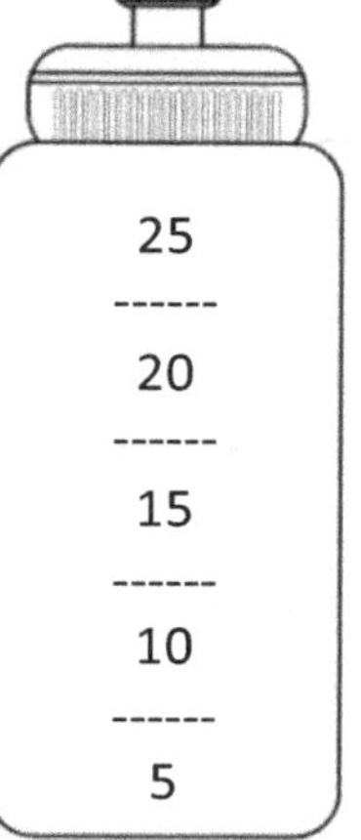

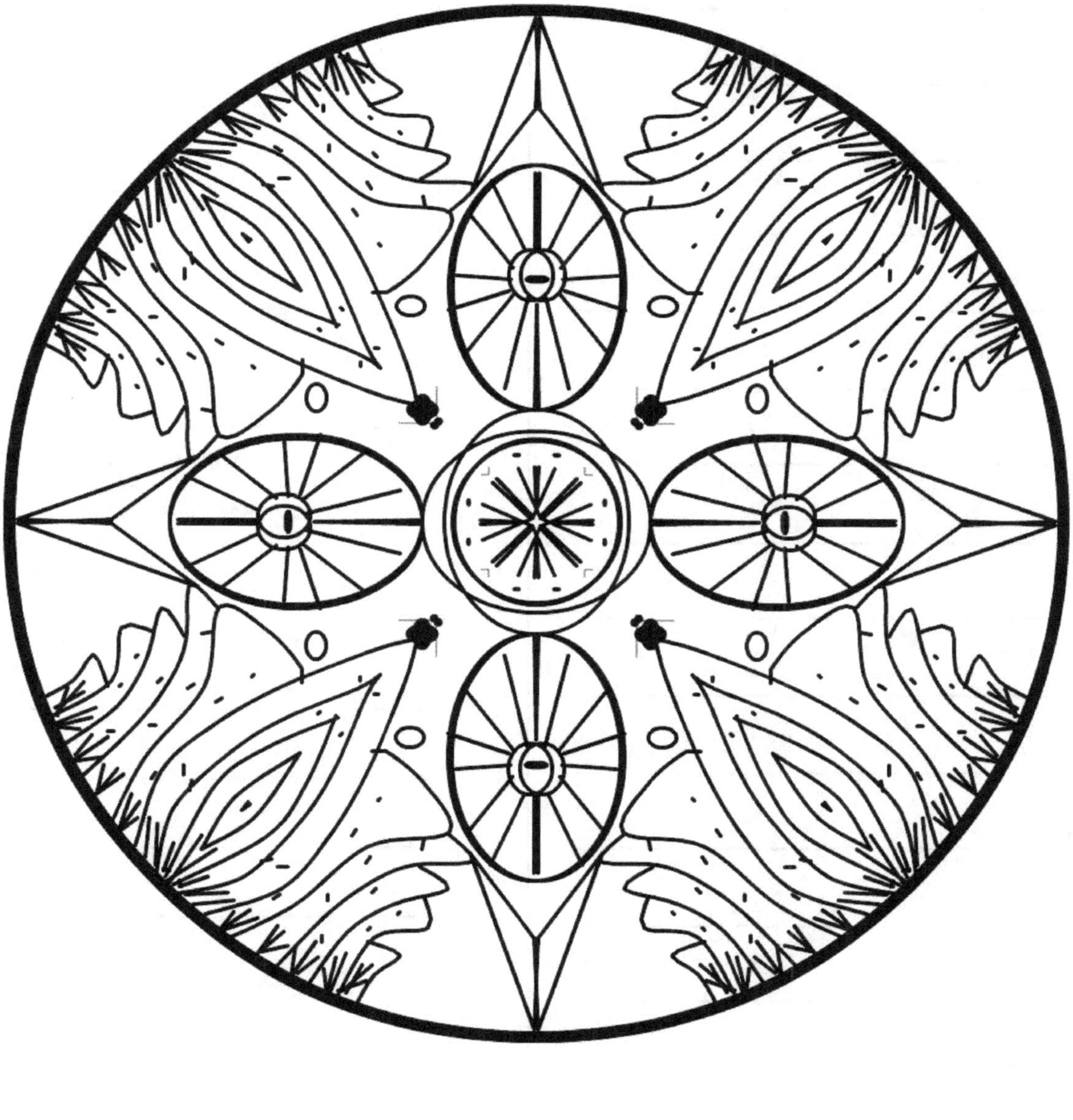

25
20
15
10
5

Day Twelve ______

5:00 ______
6:00 ______
7:00 ______
8:00 ______
9:00 ______
10:00 ______
11:00 ______
Noon ______
1:00 ______
2:00 ______
3:00 ______
4:00 ______
5:00 ______
6:00 ______
7:00 ______
8:00 ______
9:00 ______
10:00 ______
11:00 ______
Midnight ______

top priorities for today

______
______
______
______
______

Today's victories

List 4 ways you show compassion.

______
______
______
______
______
______
______
______

The Stella Society Training

Exercise	Set 1	Set 2	Set 3	Set 4	Set 5	notes

Time started: ____________ Time ended: ____________

Location: ____

Feelings before training:

Feelings after training

NUTRITION

Meal 1

time eaten: _________

Meal 2

time eaten: _________

Meal 3

time eaten: _________

Meal 4

time eaten: _________

Meal 5

time eaten: _________

Hydration

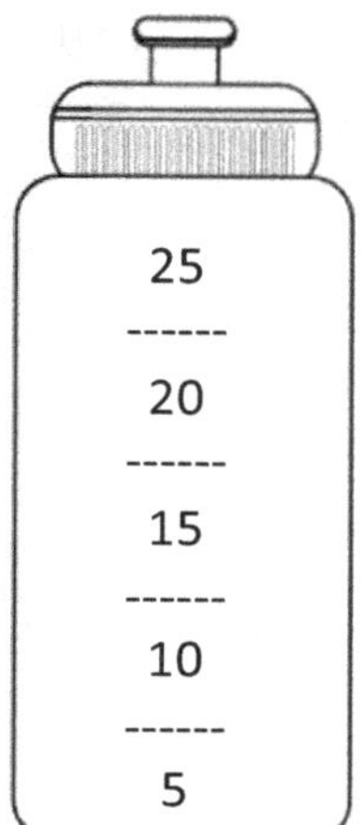

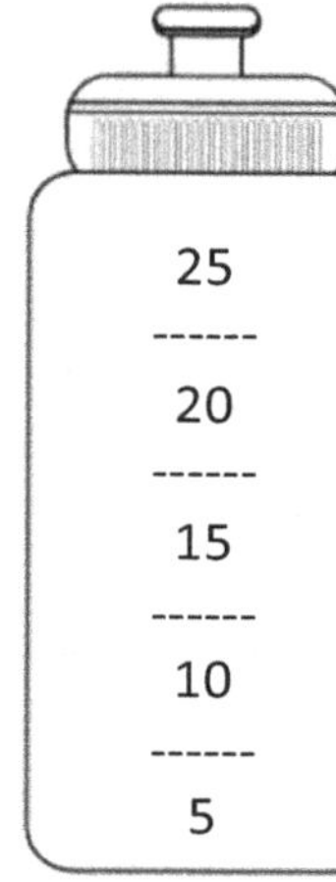

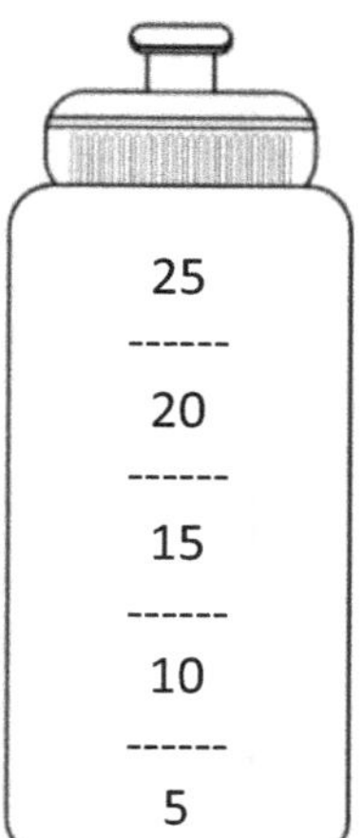

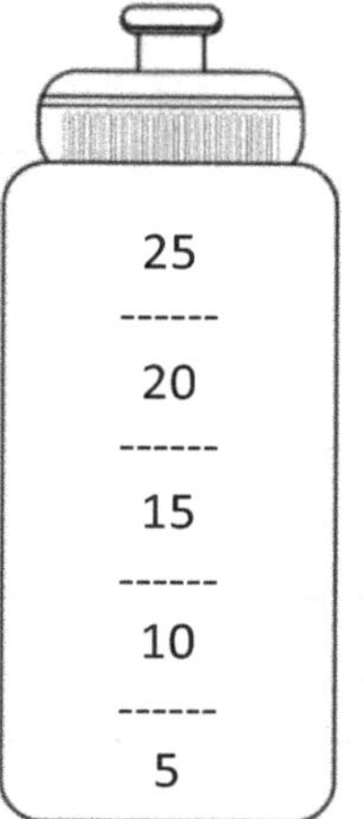

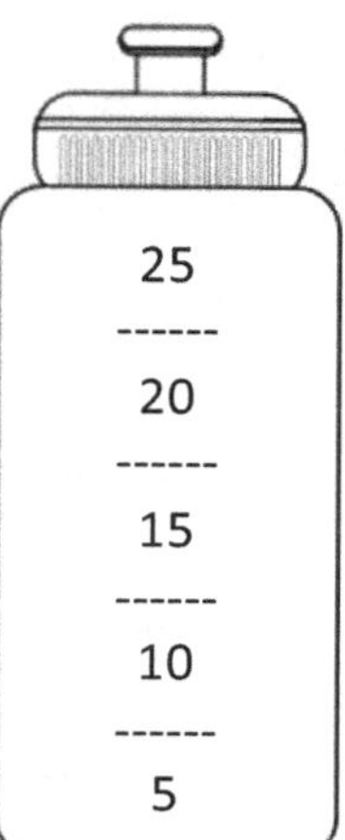

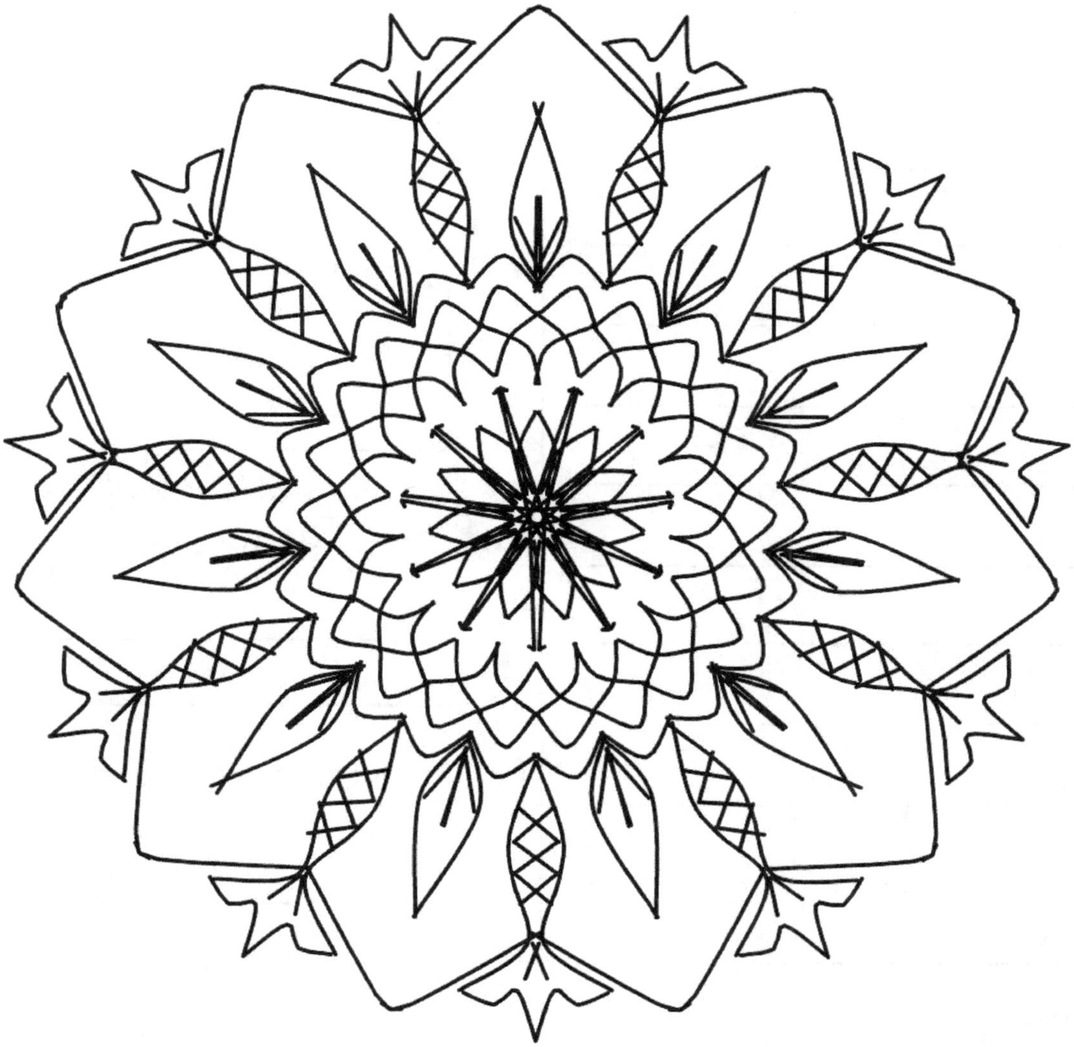

Day Thirteen ______

5:00 ____________________
6:00 ____________________
7:00 ____________________
8:00 ____________________
9:00 ____________________
10:00 ____________________
11:00 ____________________
Noon ____________________
1:00 ____________________
2:00 ____________________
3:00 ____________________
4:00 ____________________
5:00 ____________________
6:00 ____________________
7:00 ____________________
8:00 ____________________
9:00 ____________________
10:00 ____________________
11:00 ____________________
Midnight ____________________

top priorities for today

____
____
____
____

Today's victories

Who needs roses from your garden and why?

____
____
____
____
____
____
____

The Stella Society Training

Exercise	Set 1	Set 2	Set 3	Set 4	Set 5	notes

Time started: ____________ Time ended: _____________

Location: ____

Feelings before training:

Feelings after training

NUTRITION

Meal 1

time eaten: _________

Meal 2

time eaten: _________

Meal 3

time eaten: _________

Meal 4

time eaten: _________

Meal 5

time eaten: _________

Hydration

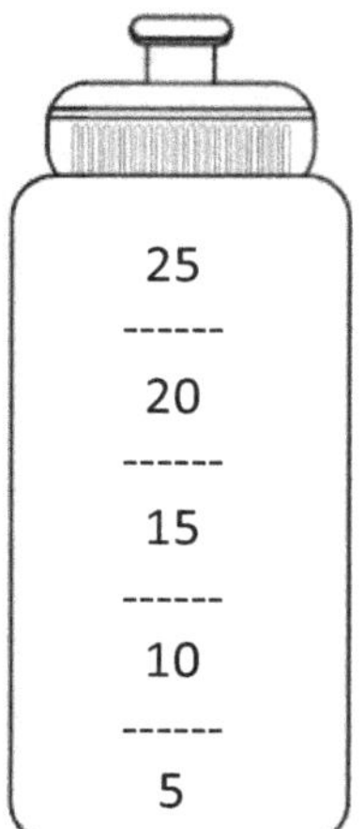

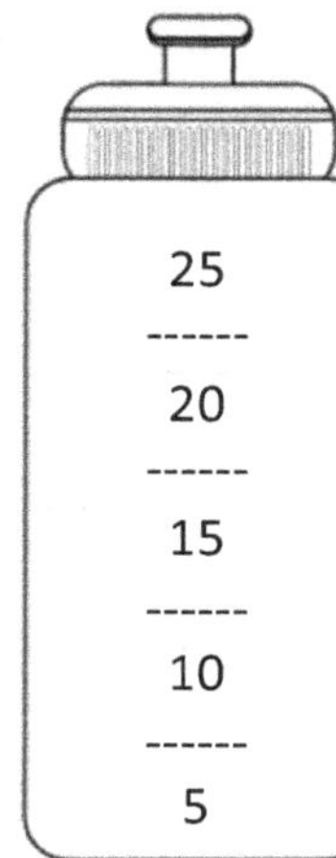

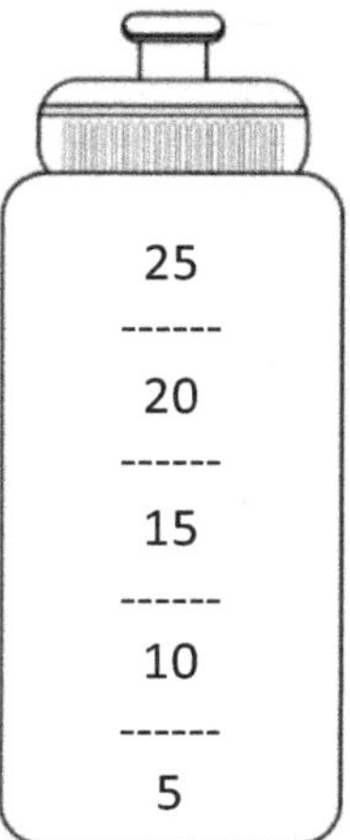

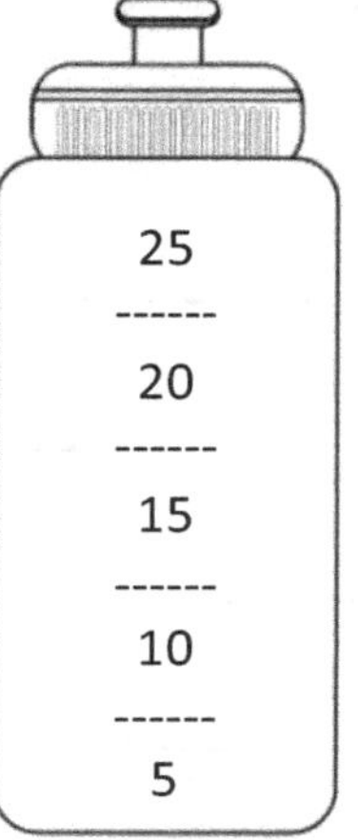

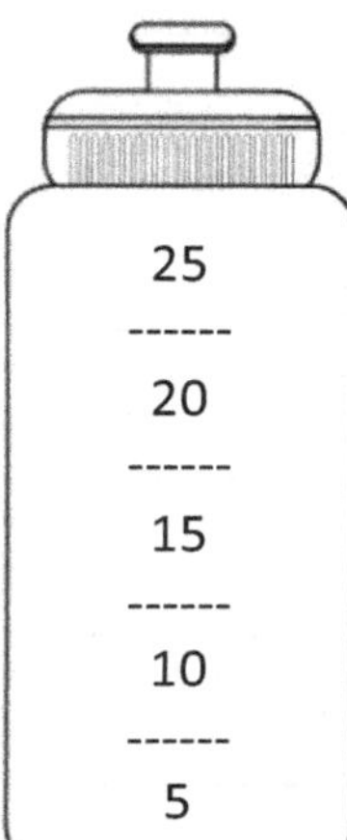

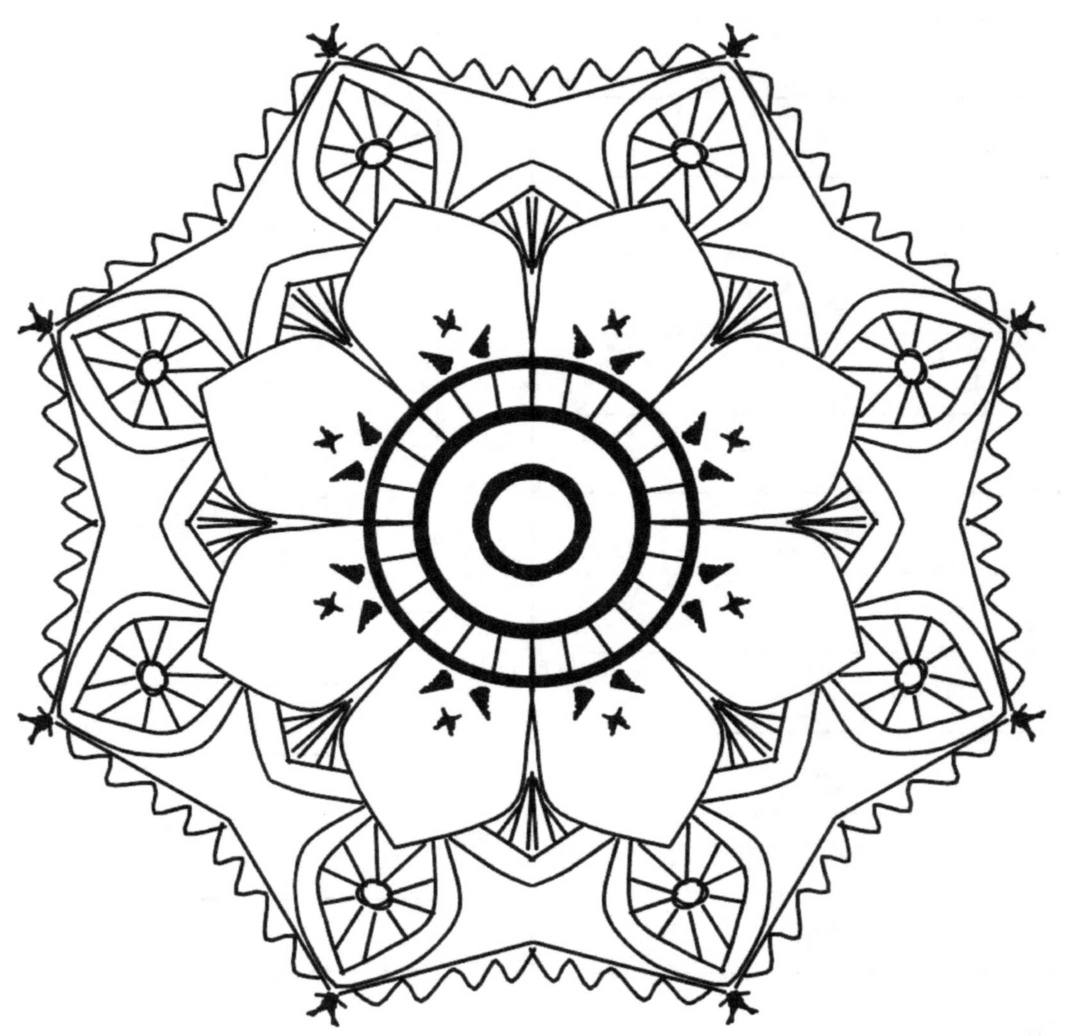

Day Fourteen ______

5:00 ______

6:00 ______

7:00 ______

8:00 ______

9:00 ______

10:00 ______

11:00 ______

Noon ______

1:00 ______

2:00 ______

3:00 ______

4:00 ______

5:00 ______

6:00 ______

7:00 ______

8:00 ______

9:00 ______

10:00 ______

11:00 ______

Midnight ______

top priorities for today

______

______

______

______

______

Today's victories

What should you forgive your self for?

______

______

______

______

______

______

______

______

BE FORGIVING

The Stella Society Training

Exercise	Set 1	Set 2	Set 3	Set 4	Set 5	notes

Time started: ____________ Time ended: ______________

Location: ____

Feelings before training:

Feelings after training

NUTRITION

Meal 1

time eaten: _________

Meal 2

time eaten: _________

Meal 3

time eaten: _________

Meal 4

time eaten: _________

Meal 5

time eaten: _________

Hydration

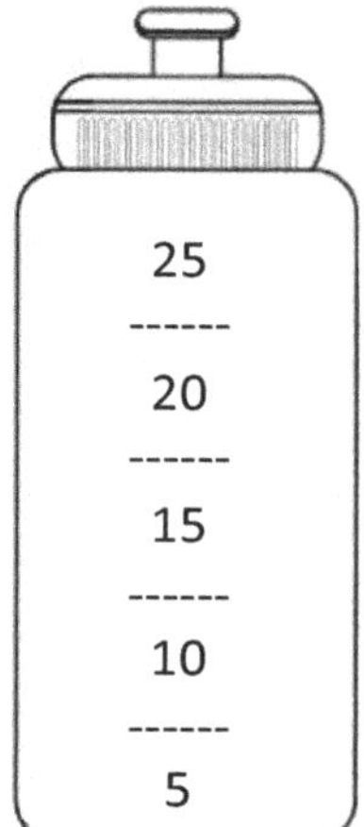

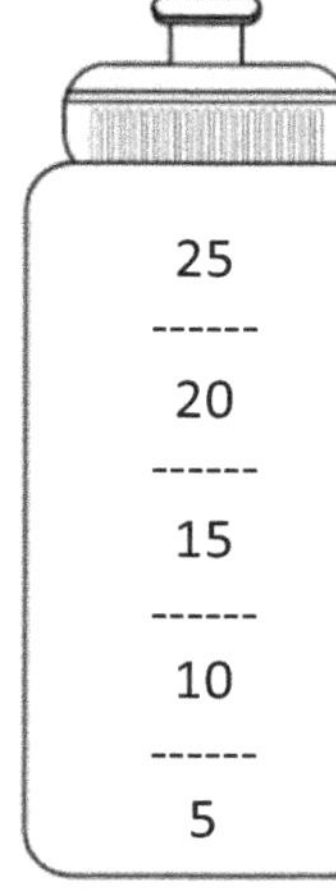

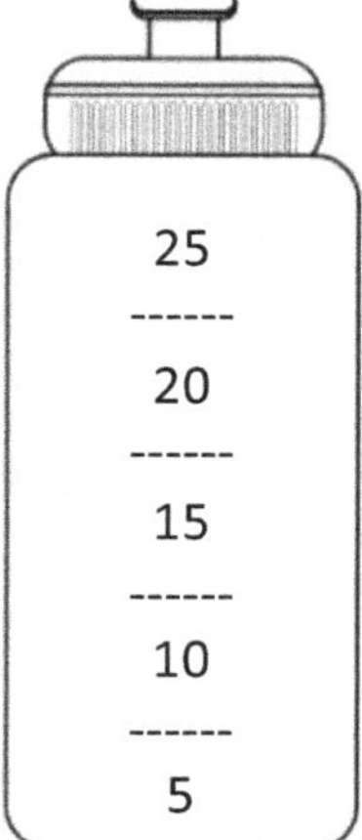

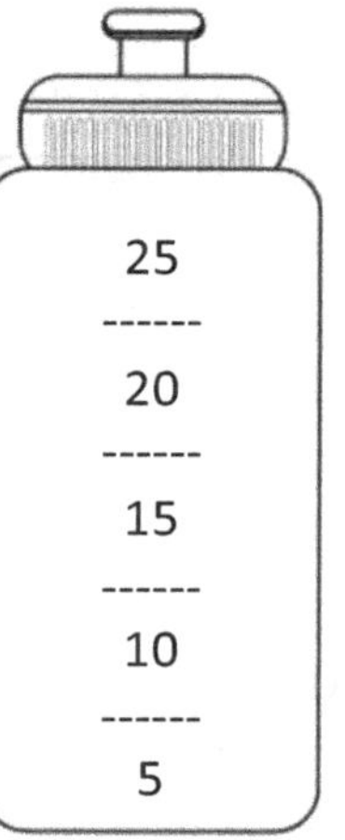

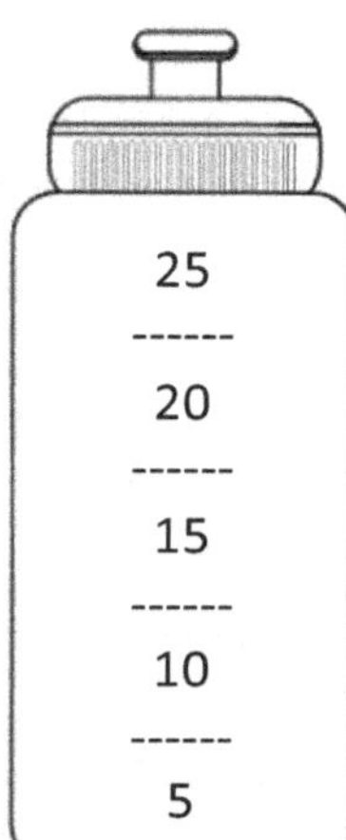

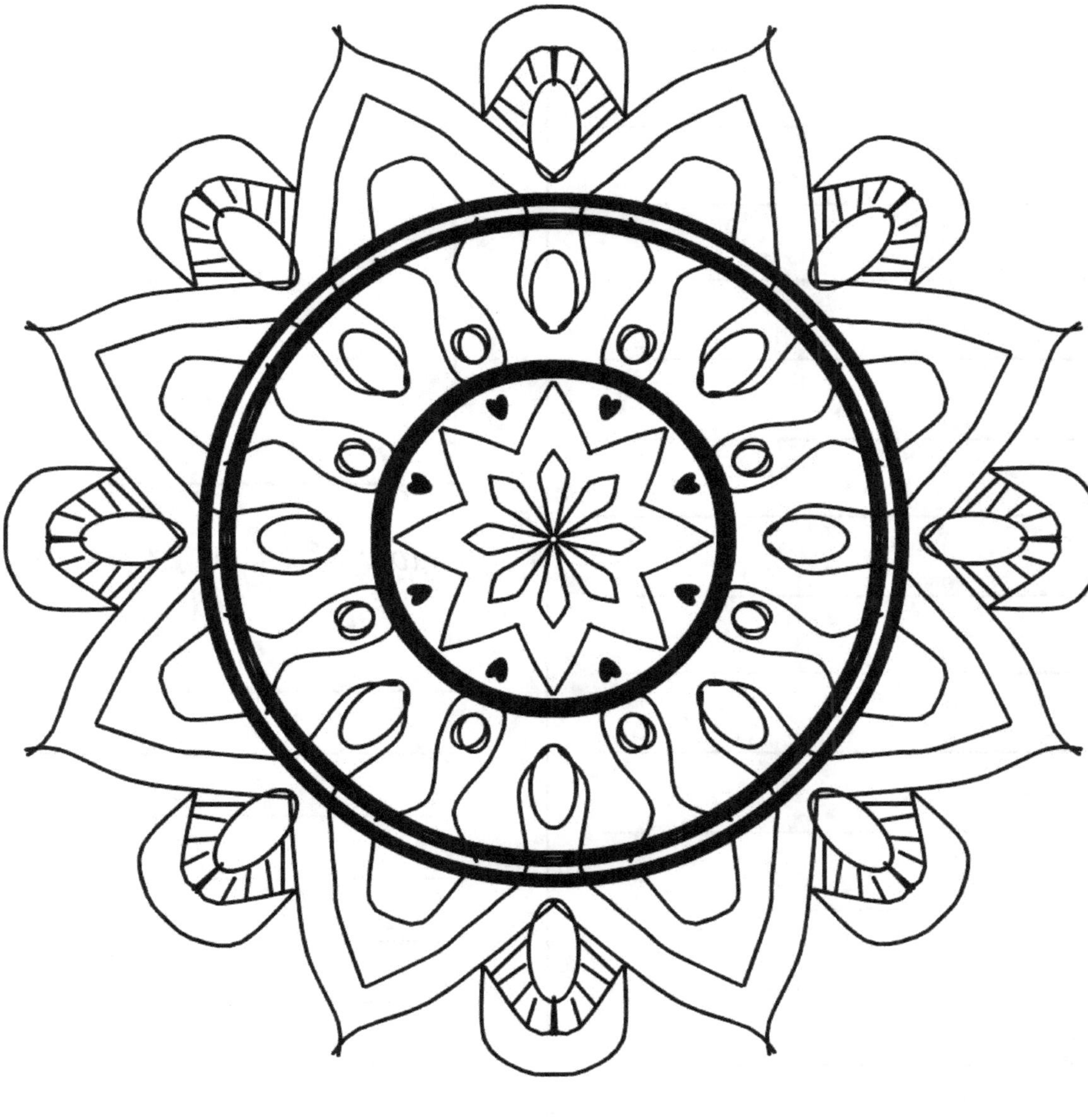

Day Fifteen ______

5:00 ______

6:00 ______

7:00 ______

8:00 ______

9:00 ______

10:00 ______

11:00 ______

Noon ______

1:00 ______

2:00 ______

3:00 ______

4:00 ______

5:00 ______

6:00 ______

7:00 ______

8:00 ______

9:00 ______

10:00 ______

11:00 ______

Midnight ______

top priorities for today

Today's victories

How will you be remarkable today?

The Stella Society Training

Exercise	Set 1	Set 2	Set 3	Set 4	Set 5	notes

Time started: ____________ Time ended: _____________

Location: ____

Feelings before training:

Feelings after training

NUTRITION

Meal 1

time eaten: _________

Meal 2

time eaten: _________

Meal 3

time eaten: _________

Meal 4

time eaten: _________

Meal 5

time eaten: _________

Hydration

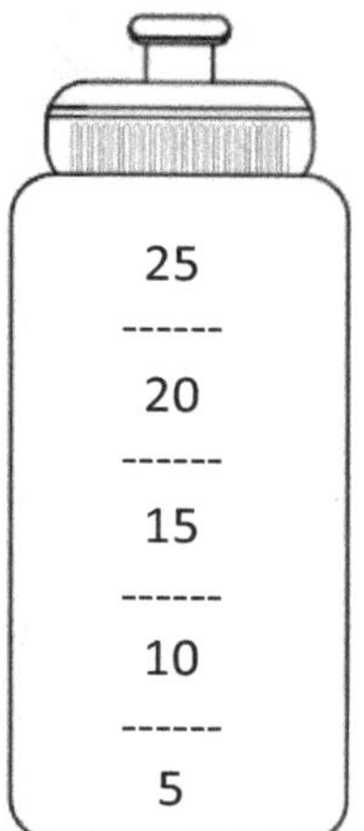

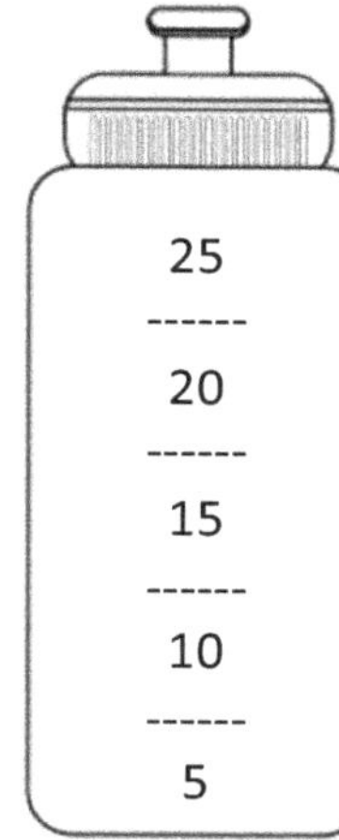

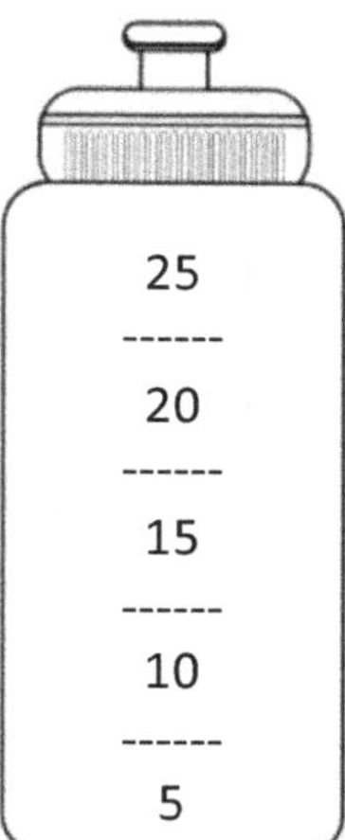

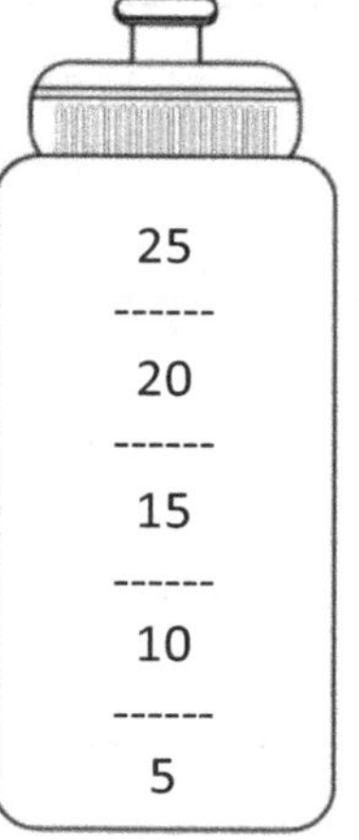

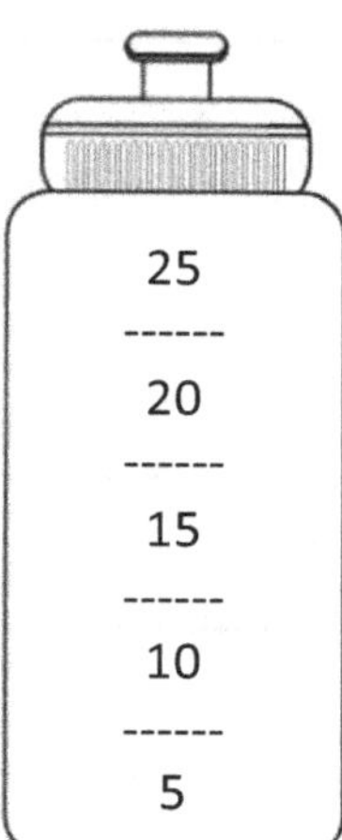

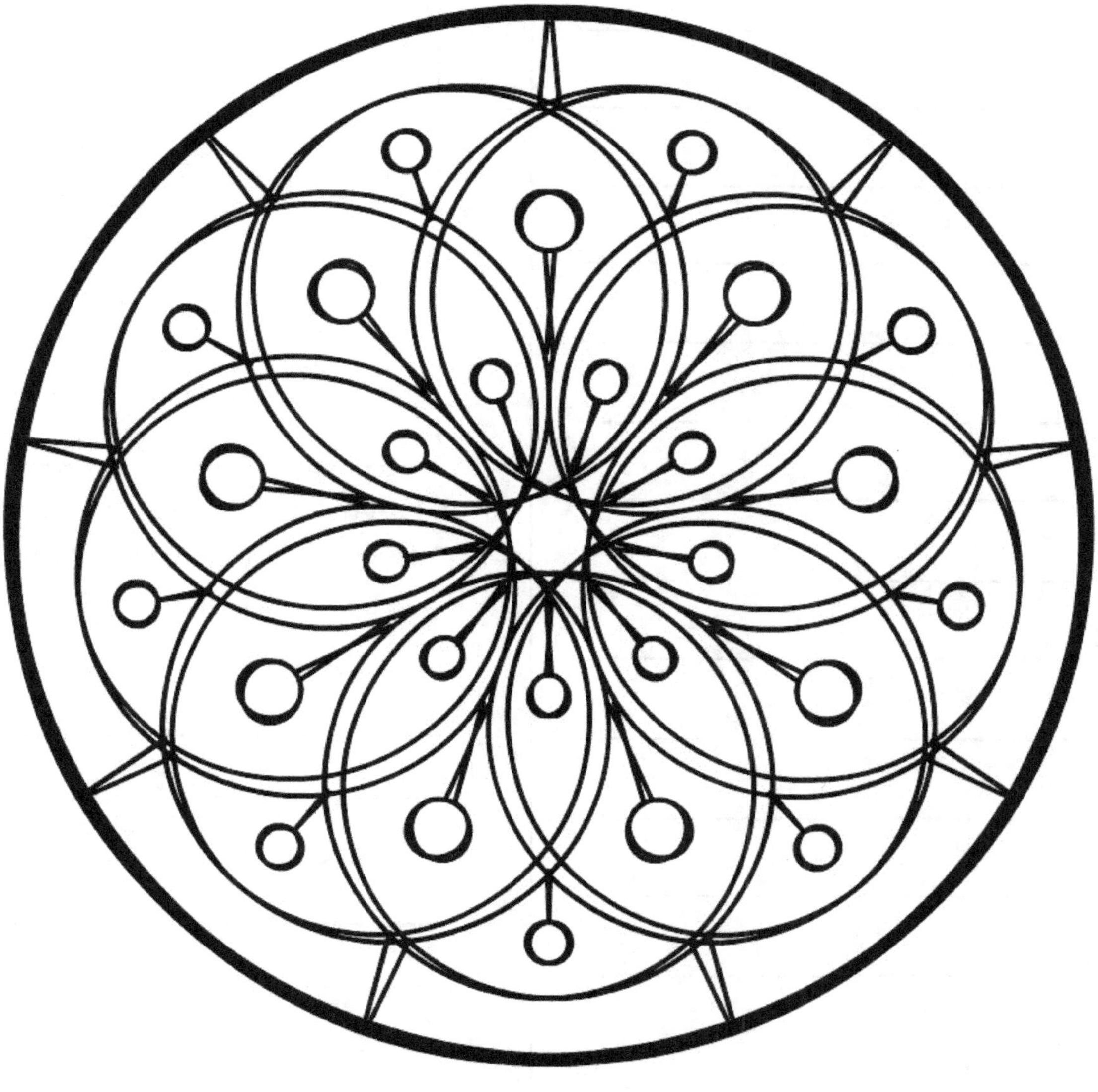

Day Sixteen ______

5:00 ______

6:00 ______

7:00 ______

8:00 ______

9:00 ______

10:00 ______

11:00 ______

Noon ______

1:00 ______

2:00 ______

3:00 ______

4:00 ______

5:00 ______

6:00 ______

7:00 ______

8:00 ______

9:00 ______

10:00 ______

11:00 ______

Midnight ______

top priorities for today

______

______

______

______

______

Today's victories

Watch the sunset and list 5 places you want to see it happen?

______

______

______

______

______

______

______

______

The Stella Society Training

Exercise	Set 1	Set 2	Set 3	Set 4	Set 5	notes

Time started: ____________ Time ended: _____________

Location: ____

Feelings before training: 🙂 😑 ☹️ 😝 😠 😕 😇 😎

Feelings after training 🙂 😑 ☹️ 😝 😠 😕 😇 😎

NUTRITION

Meal 1

time eaten: _________

Meal 2

time eaten: _________

Meal 3

time eaten: _________

Meal 4

time eaten: _________

Meal 5

time eaten: _________

Hydration

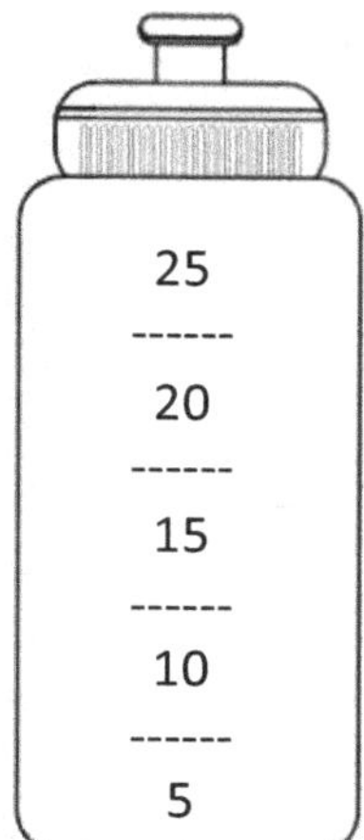

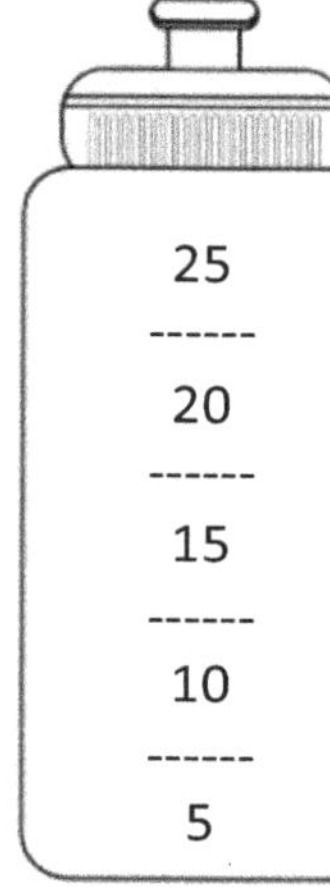

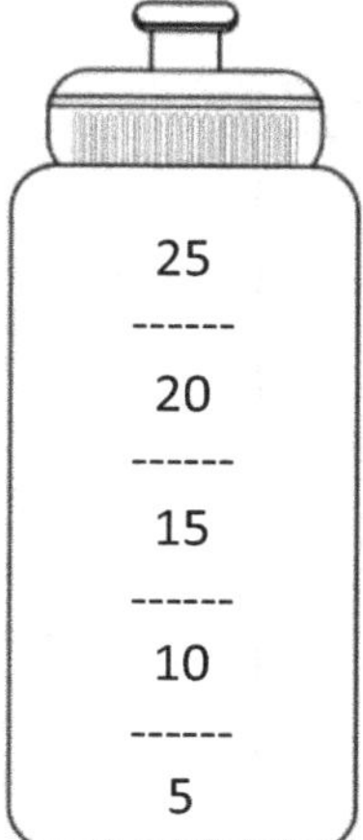

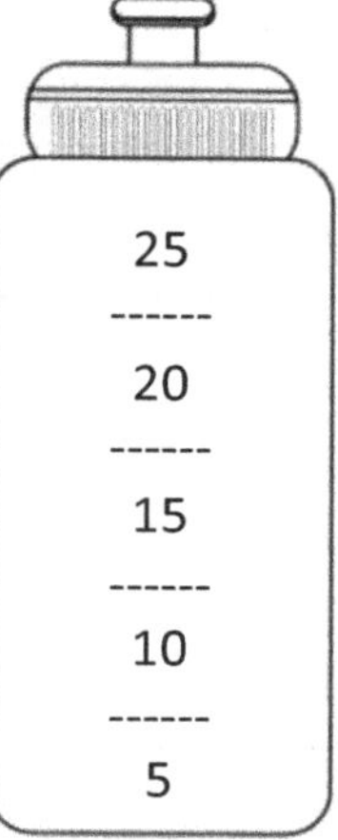

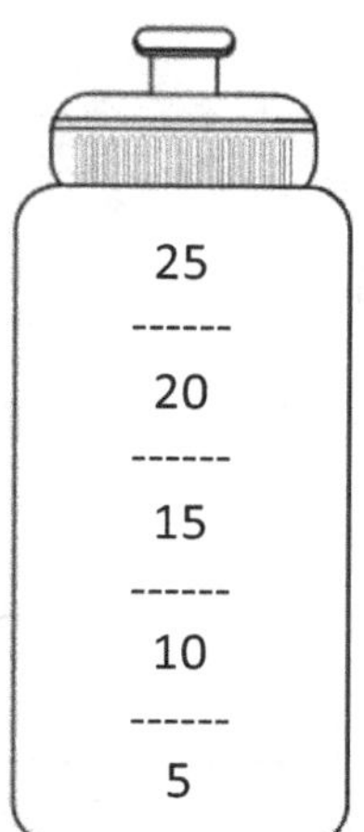

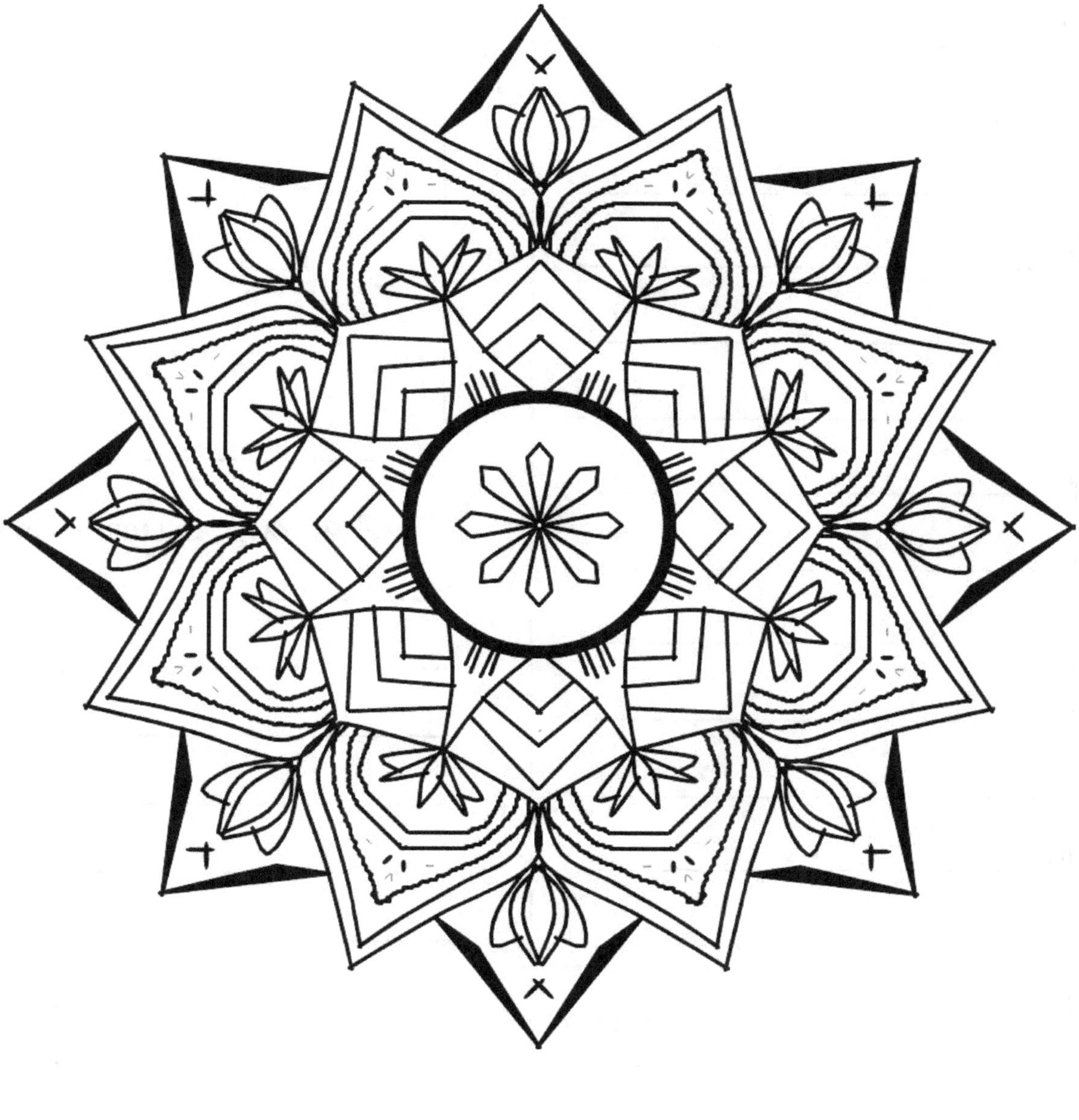

Day Seventeen ______

5:00 ____________________
6:00 ____________________
7:00 ____________________
8:00 ____________________
9:00 ____________________
10:00 ____________________
11:00 ____________________
Noon ____________________
1:00 ____________________
2:00 ____________________
3:00 ____________________
4:00 ____________________
5:00 ____________________
6:00 ____________________
7:00 ____________________
8:00 ____________________
9:00 ____________________
10:00 ____________________
11:00 ____________________
Midnight ____________________

top priorities for today

____
____
____
____
____

Today's victories

What makes you happy?

____
____
____
____
____
____
____
____

The Stella Society Training

Exercise	Set 1	Set 2	Set 3	Set 4	Set 5	notes

Time started: ____________ Time ended: _____________

Location: ____

Feelings before training:

Feelings after training

NUTRITION

Meal 1

time eaten: _________

Meal 2

time eaten: _________

Meal 3

time eaten: _________

Meal 4

time eaten: _________

Meal 5

time eaten: _________

Hydration

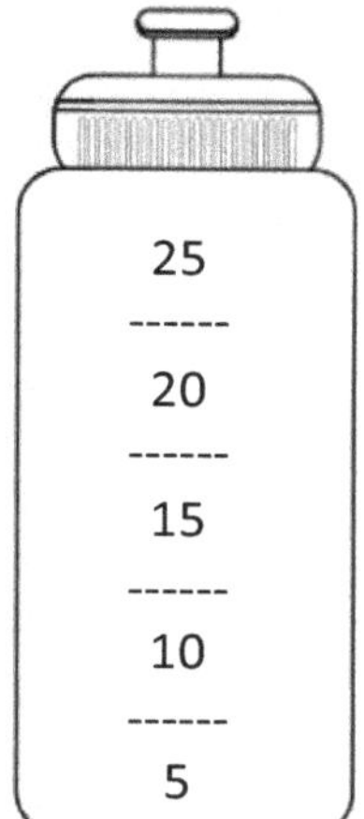

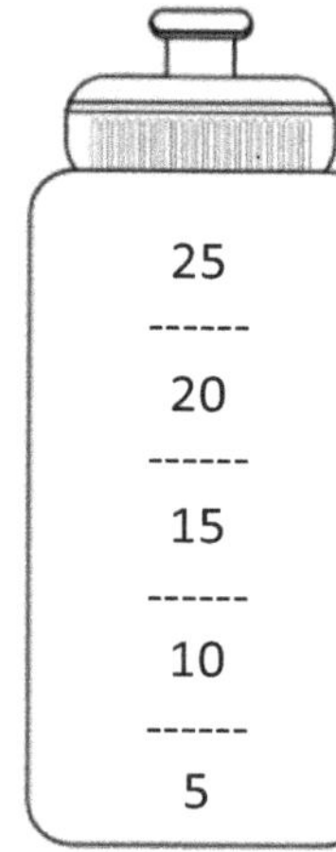

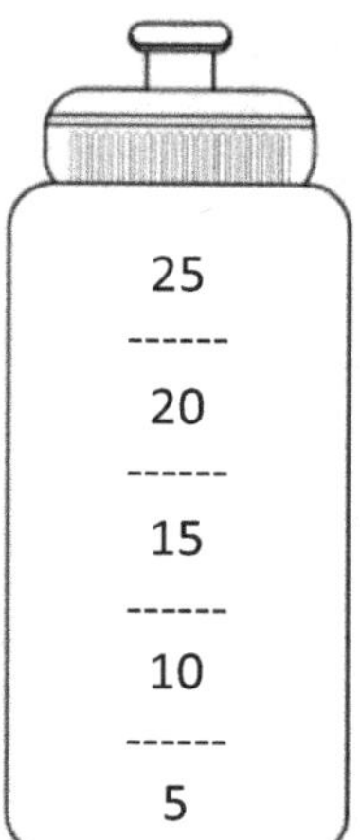

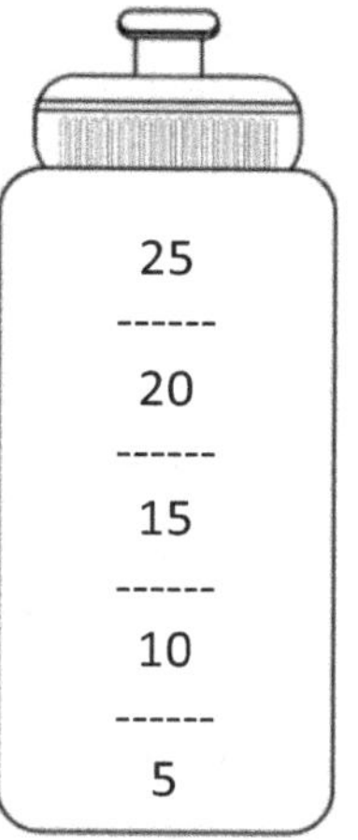

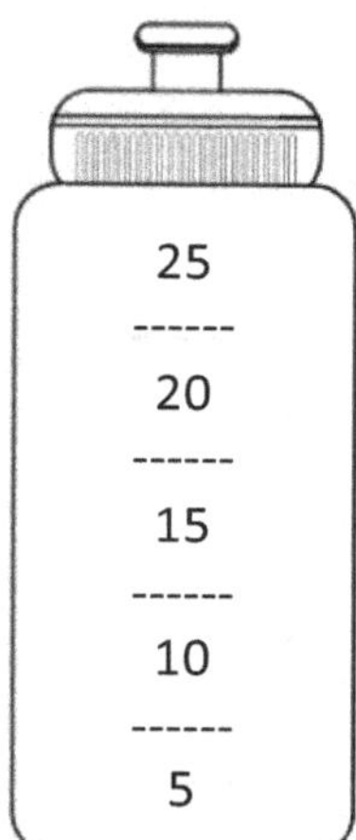

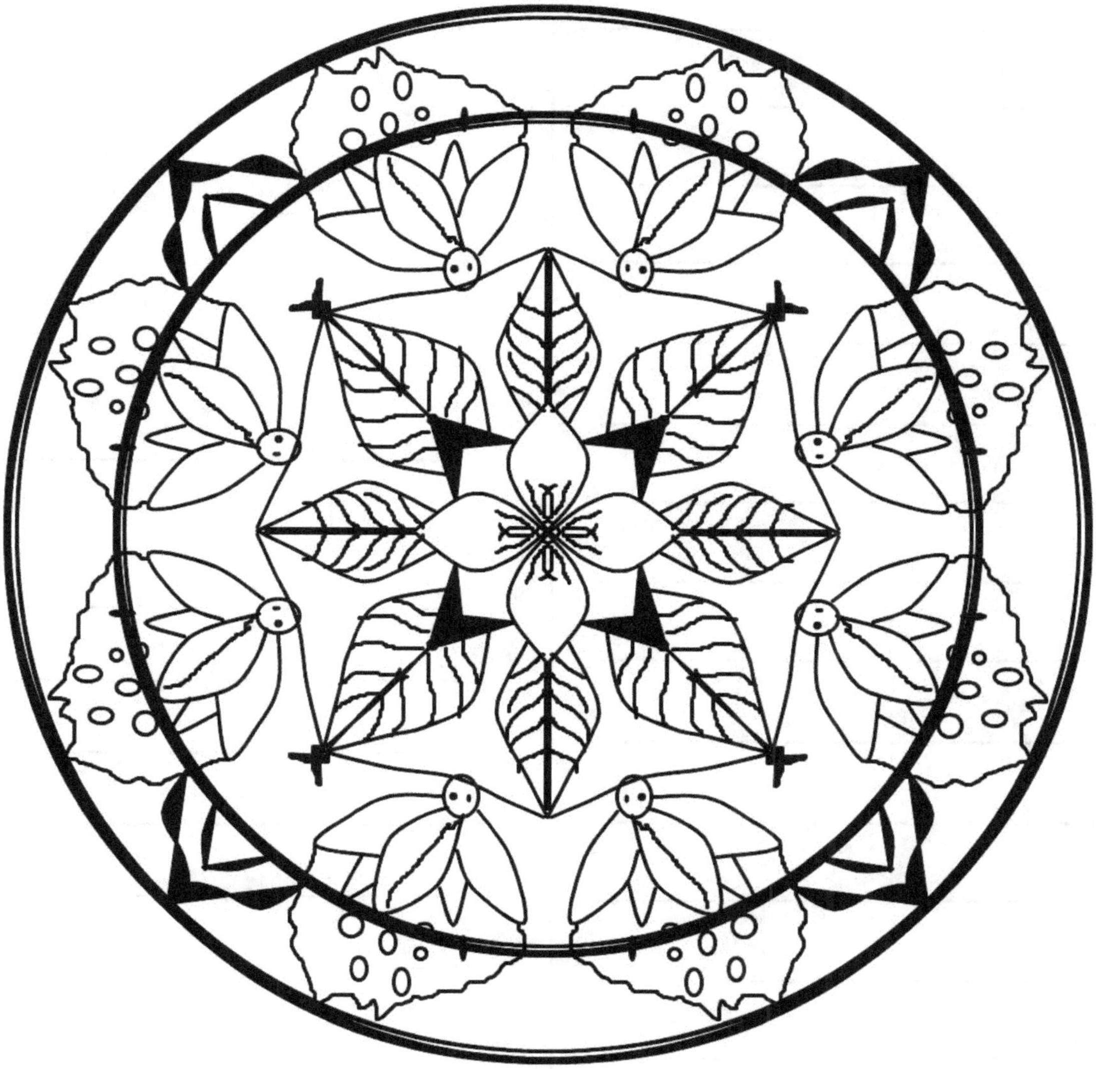

Day Eighteen ______

5:00 ______
6:00 ______
7:00 ______
8:00 ______
9:00 ______
10:00 ______
11:00 ______
Noon ______
1:00 ______
2:00 ______
3:00 ______
4:00 ______
5:00 ______
6:00 ______
7:00 ______
8:00 ______
9:00 ______
10:00 ______
11:00 ______
Midnight ______

top priorities for today

______
______
______
______
______

Today's victories

Where will you shine your light this week?

______
______
______
______
______
______
______
______

The Stella Society Training

Exercise	Set 1	Set 2	Set 3	Set 4	Set 5	notes

Time started: ____________ Time ended: _____________

Location: ____

Feelings before training: ☺ 😑 ☹ 😝 😠 😕 😇 😎

Feelings after training ☺ 😑 ☹ 😝 😠 😕 😇 😎

NUTRITION

Meal 1

time eaten: _________

Meal 2

time eaten: _________

Meal 3

time eaten: _________

Meal 4

time eaten: _________

Meal 5

time eaten: _________

Hydration

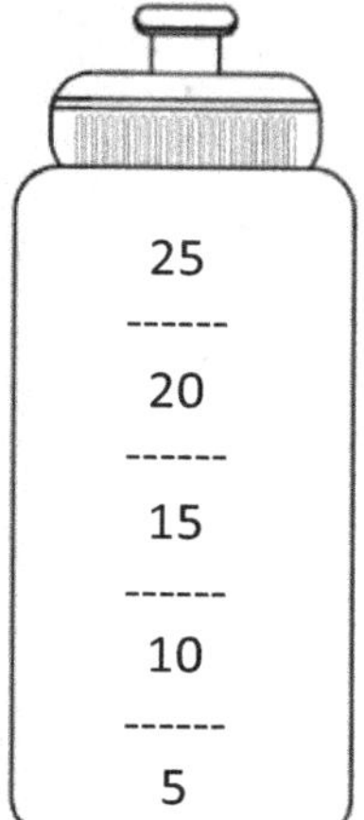

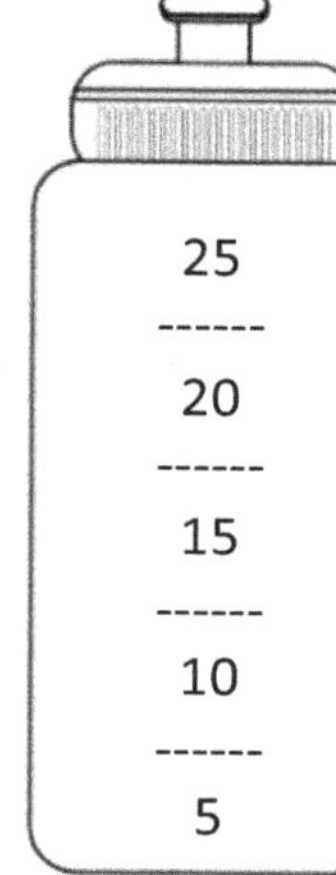

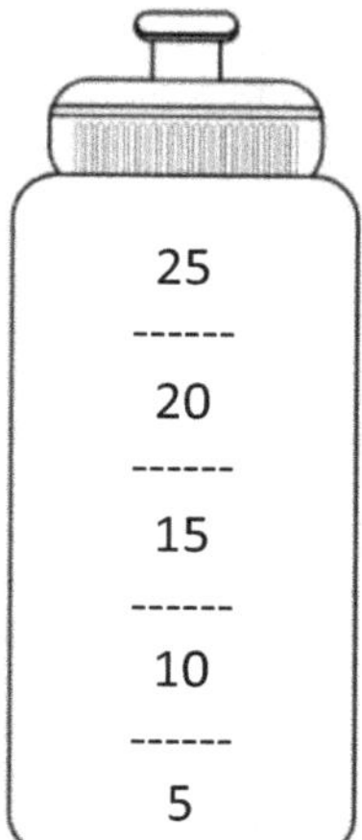

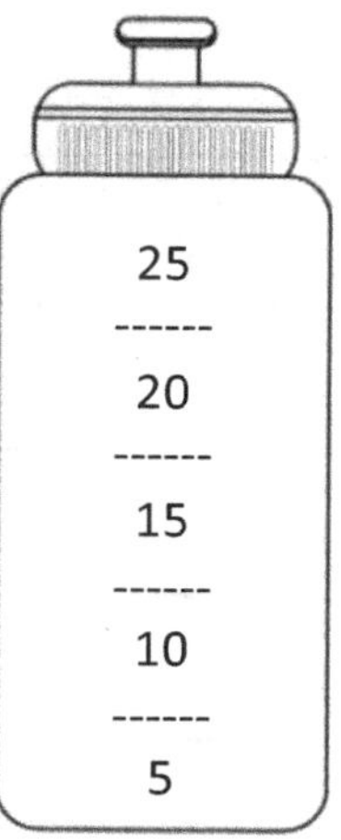

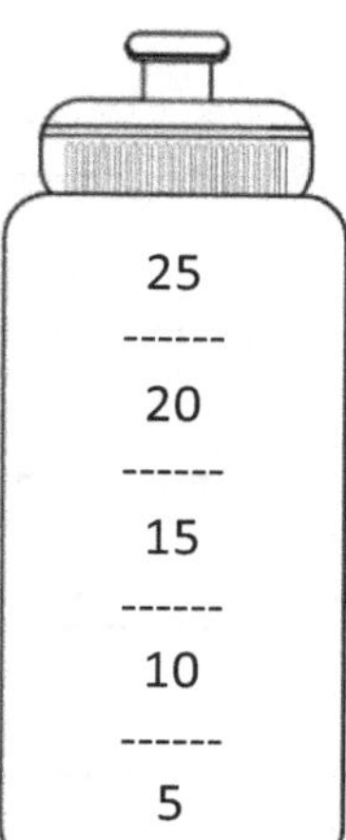

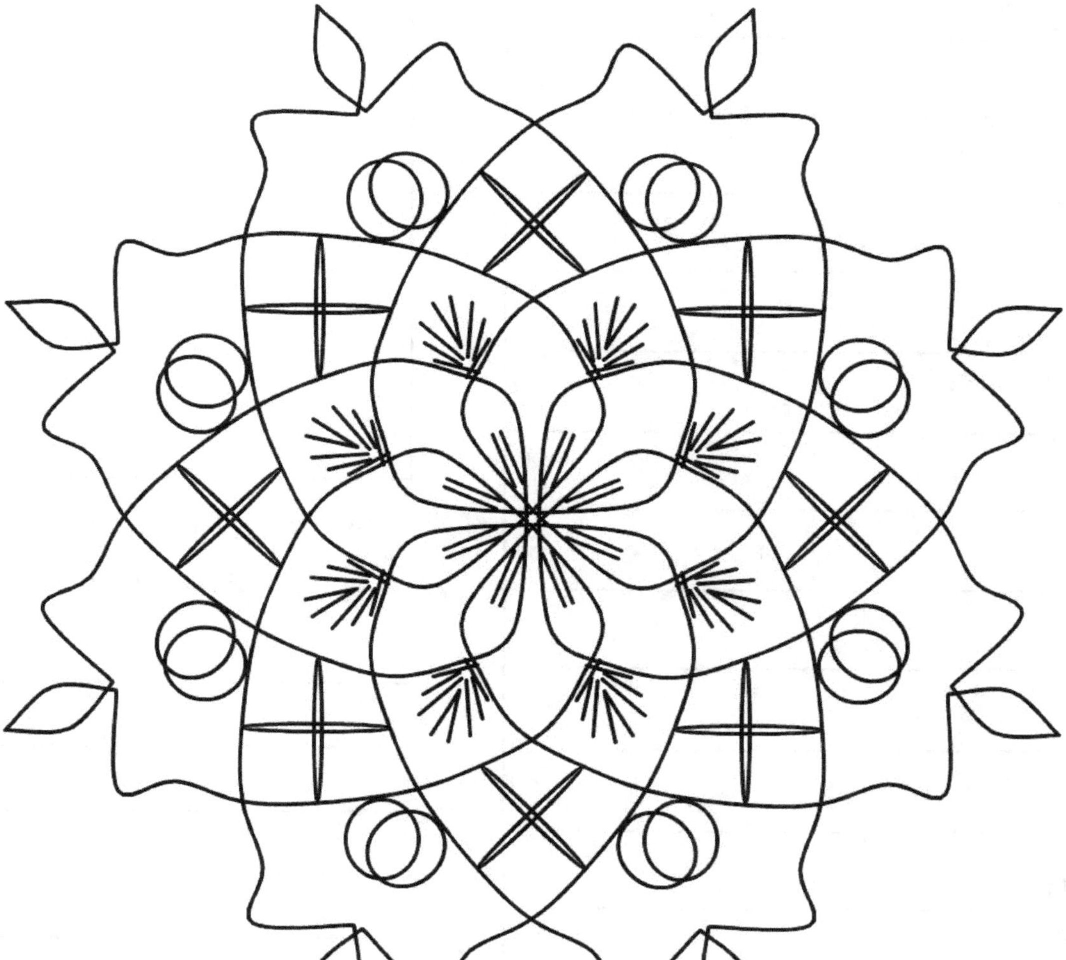

Day Nineteen ______

5:00 ______
6:00 ______
7:00 ______
8:00 ______
9:00 ______
10:00 ______
11:00 ______
Noon ______
1:00 ______
2:00 ______
3:00 ______
4:00 ______
5:00 ______
6:00 ______
7:00 ______
8:00 ______
9:00 ______
10:00 ______
11:00 ______
Midnight ______

top priorities for today

Today's victories

You are charming, how will you show it?

The Stella Society Training

Exercise	Set 1	Set 2	Set 3	Set 4	Set 5	notes

Time started: ____________ Time ended: _____________

Location: ____

Feelings before training: ☺ 😑 ☹ 😝 😠 😕 😇 😎

Feelings after training ☺ 😑 ☹ 😝 😠 😕 😇 😎

NUTRITION

Meal 1

time eaten: _________

Meal 2

time eaten: _________

Meal 3

time eaten: _________

Meal 4

time eaten: _________

Meal 5

time eaten: _________

Hydration

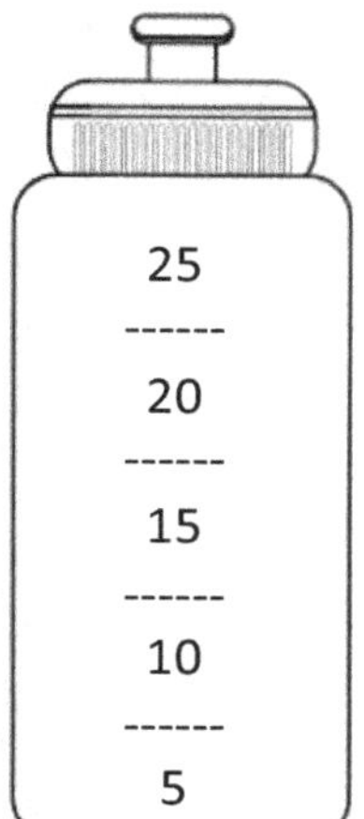

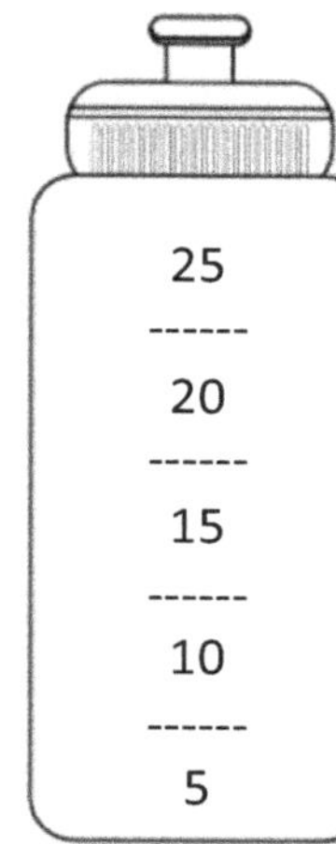

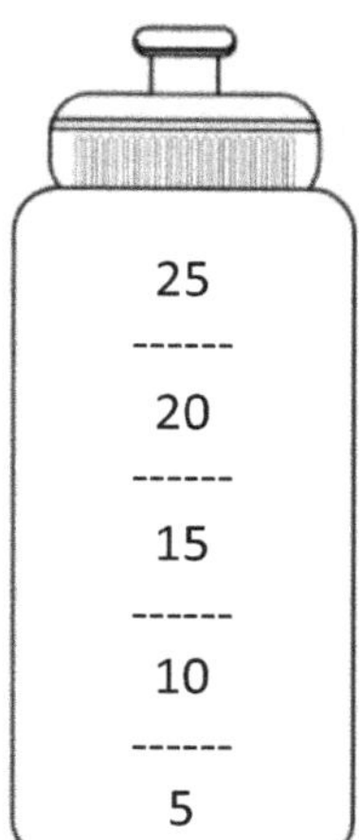

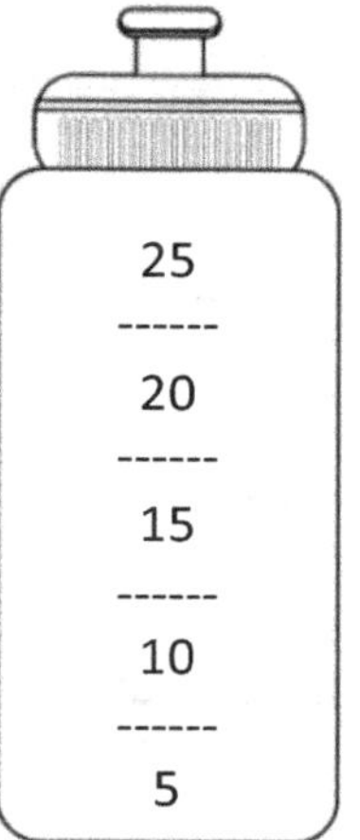

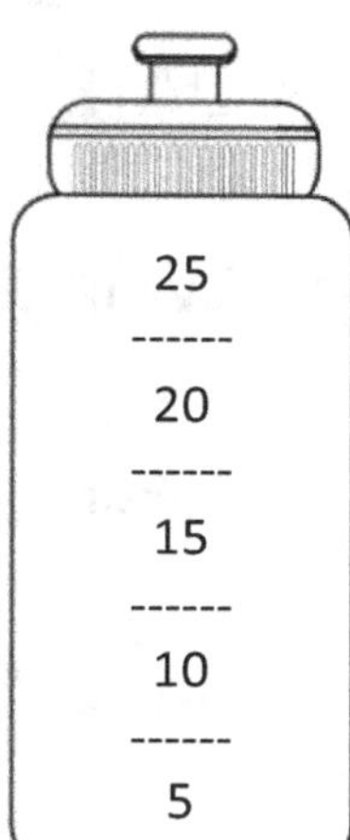

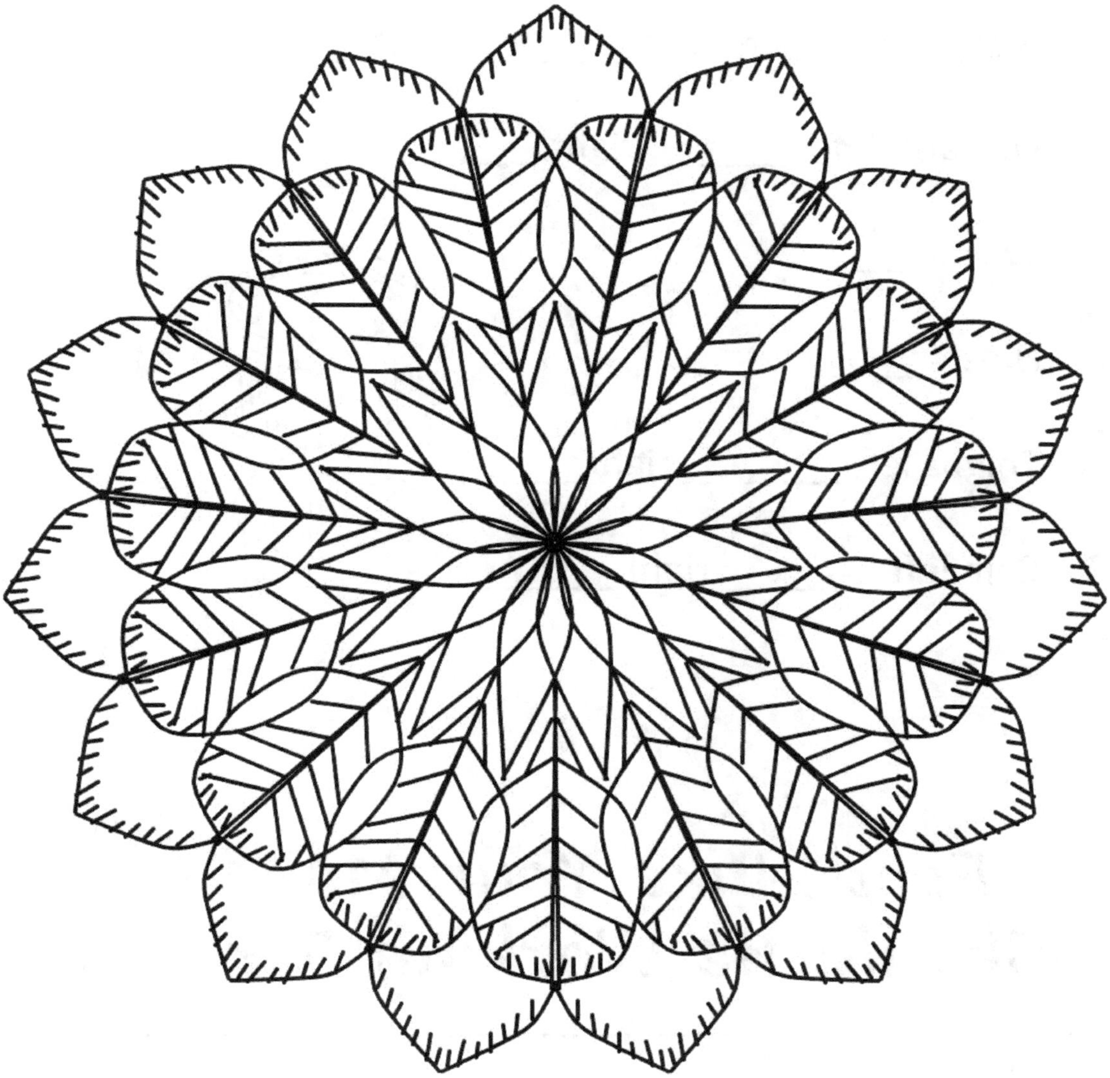

Measurements

DATE: ___________

P Weight: ______

Neck ______

R Shoulders ______

O Chest ______

Bicep / upper arm left _______ right ______

G Forearm left _______ right ______

R Waist ______

Hips ______

E Thighs left _______ right ______

S Calf left _______ right ______

S

CHECK

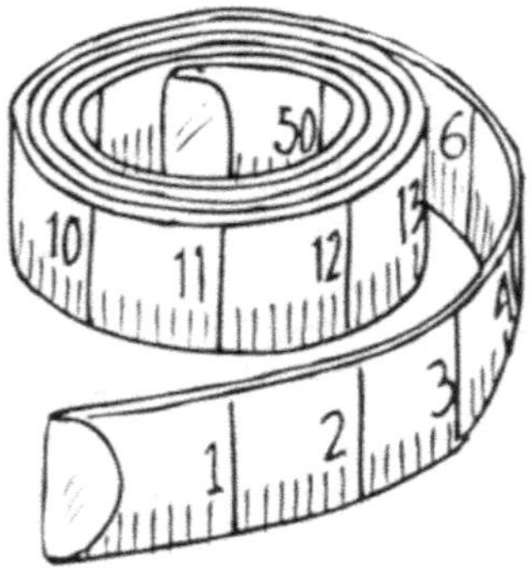

Food, Like Your Money, Should Be Working For You

Day Twenty ______

5:00 ______
6:00 ______
7:00 ______
8:00 ______
9:00 ______
10:00 ______
11:00 ______
Noon ______
1:00 ______
2:00 ______
3:00 ______
4:00 ______
5:00 ______
6:00 ______
7:00 ______
8:00 ______
9:00 ______
10:00 ______
11:00 ______
Midnight ______

top priorities for today

______
______
______
______
______

Today's victories

What is your level of understanding difficult situations?

______
______
______
______
______
______
______
______

BE UNDERSTANDING

The Stella Society Workout

Exercise	Set 1	Set 2	Set 3	Set 4	Set 5	notes

Time started: ______________ Time ended: ______________

Location: ____

Feelings before training: 😊 😑 ☹️ 😝 😠 😕 😇 😎

Feelings after training 😊 😑 ☹️ 😝 😠 😕 😇 😎

NUTRITION

Meal 1

time eaten: _________

Meal 2

time eaten: _________

Meal 3

time eaten: _________

Meal 4

time eaten: _________

Meal 5

time eaten: _________

Hydration

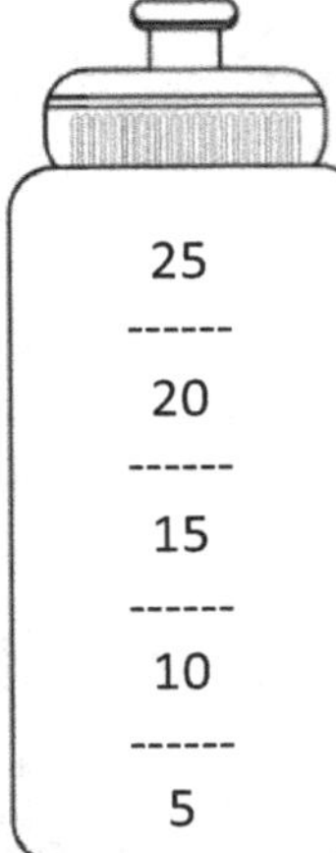

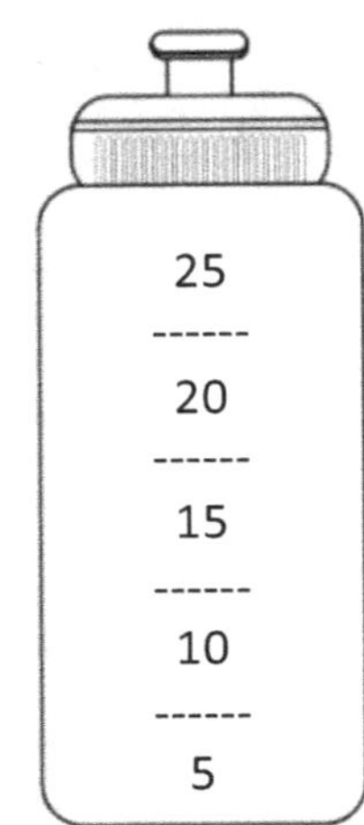

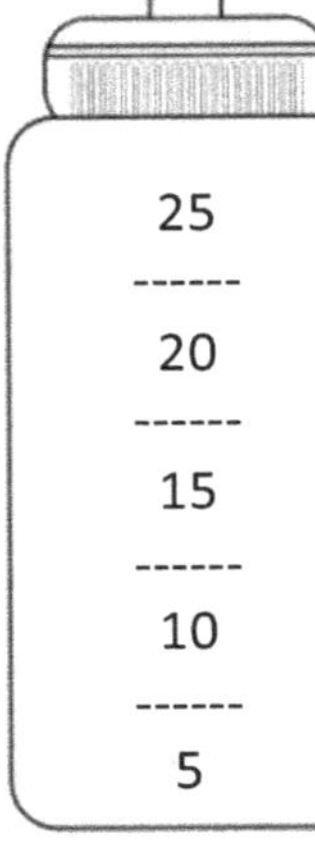

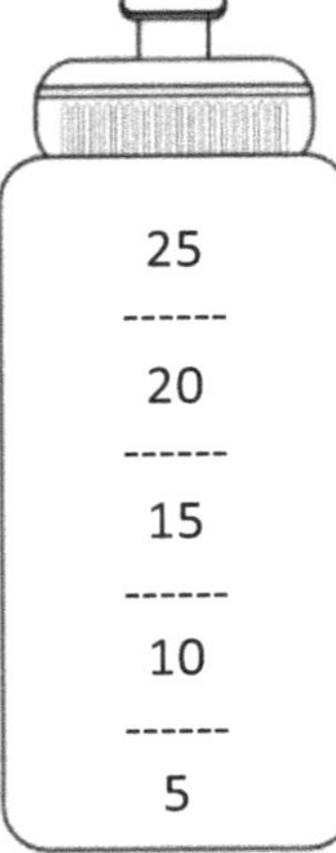

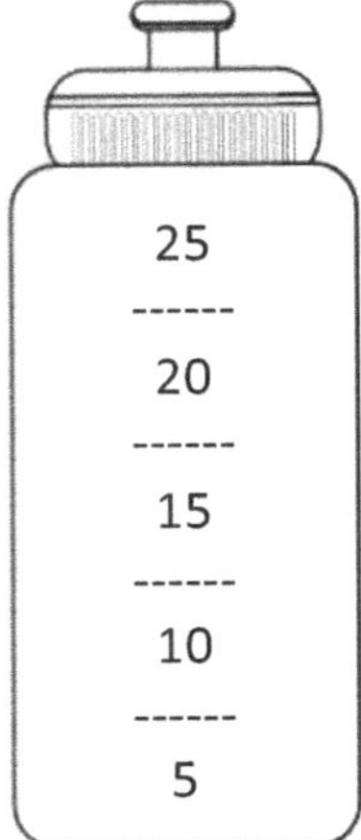

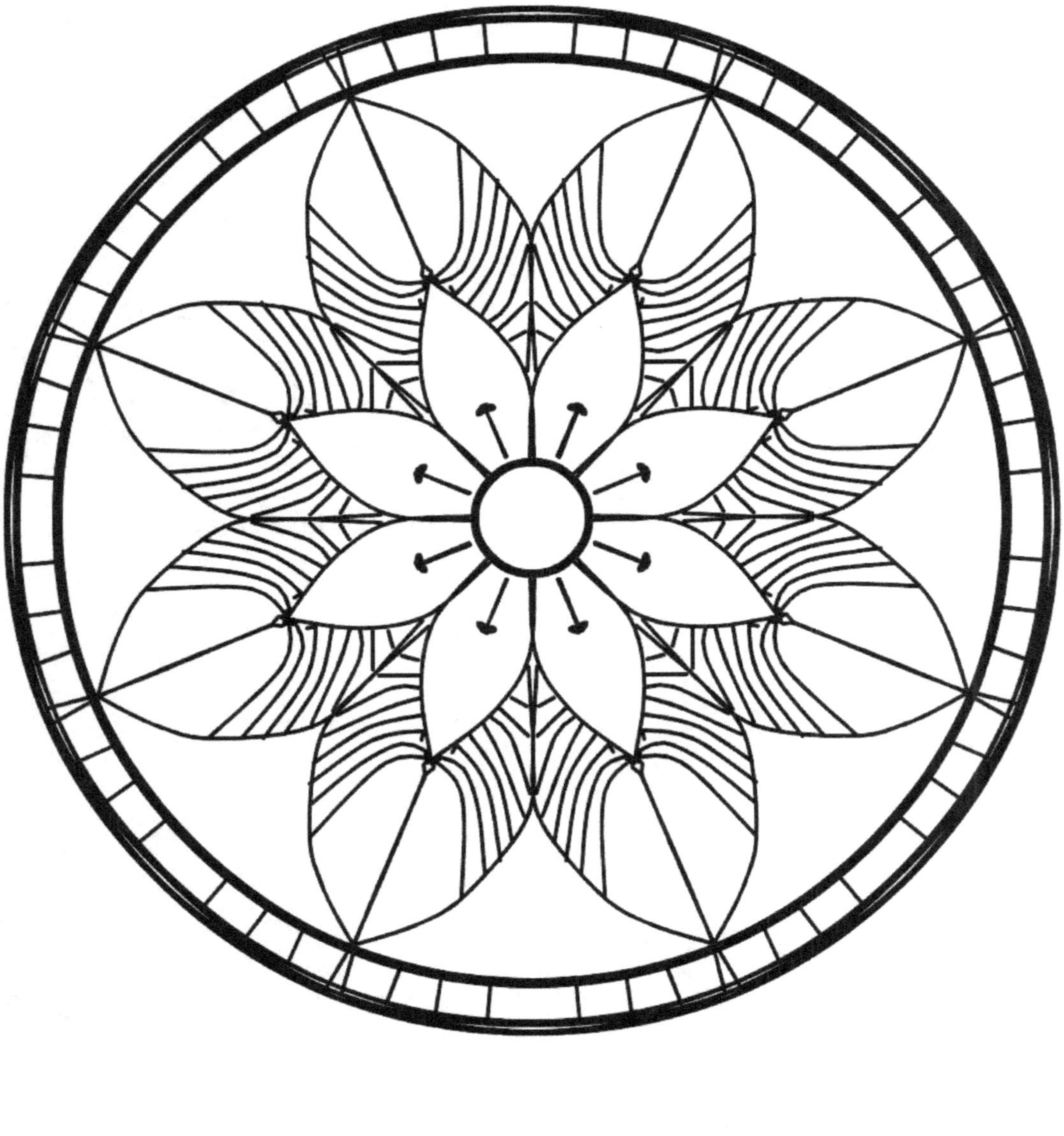

Day Twenty-one ______

5:00 ______
6:00 ______
7:00 ______
8:00 ______
9:00 ______
10:00 ______
11:00 ______
Noon ______
1:00 ______
2:00 ______
3:00 ______
4:00 ______
5:00 ______
6:00 ______
7:00 ______
8:00 ______
9:00 ______
10:00 ______
11:00 ______
Midnight ______

top priorities for today

______
______
______
______
______

Today's victories

How much can you endure?

______
______
______
______
______
______
______
______

The Stella Society Workout

Exercise	Set 1	Set 2	Set 3	Set 4	Set 5	notes

Time started: ____________ Time ended: ______________

Location: ____

Feelings before training:

Feelings after training

NUTRITION

Meal 1

time eaten: _________

Meal 2

time eaten: _________

Meal 3

time eaten: _________

Meal 4

time eaten: _________

Meal 5

time eaten: _________

Hydration

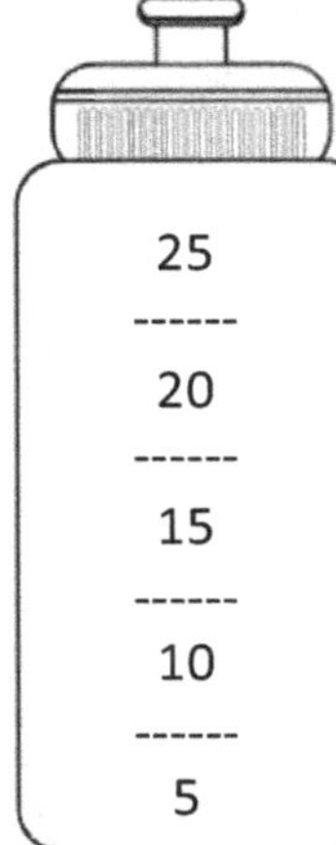

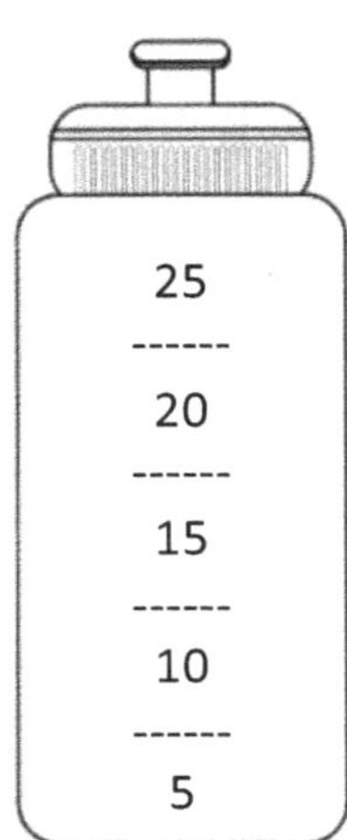

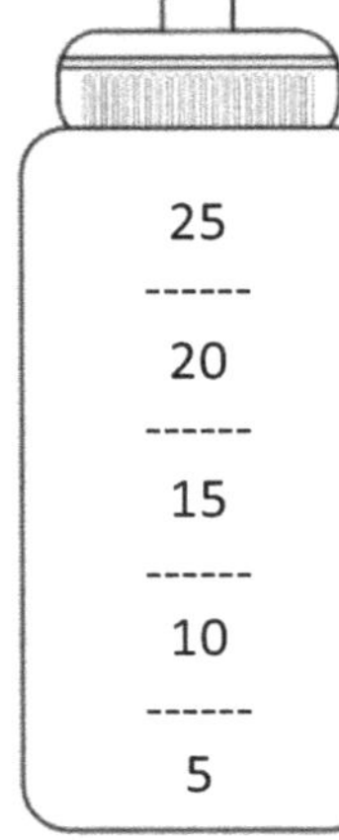

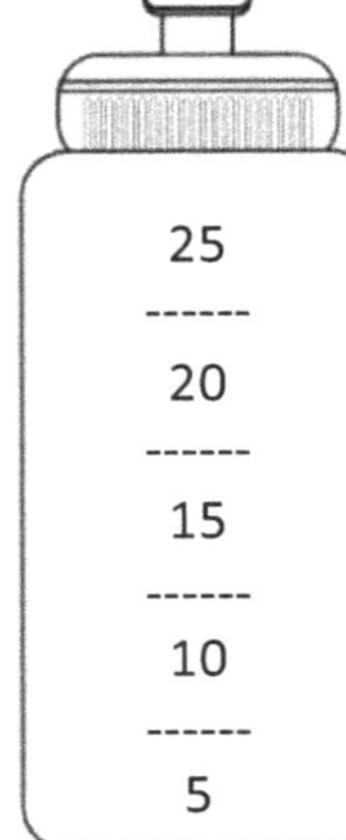

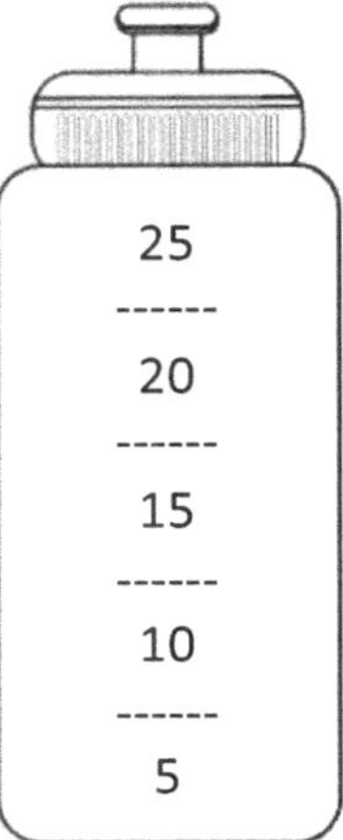

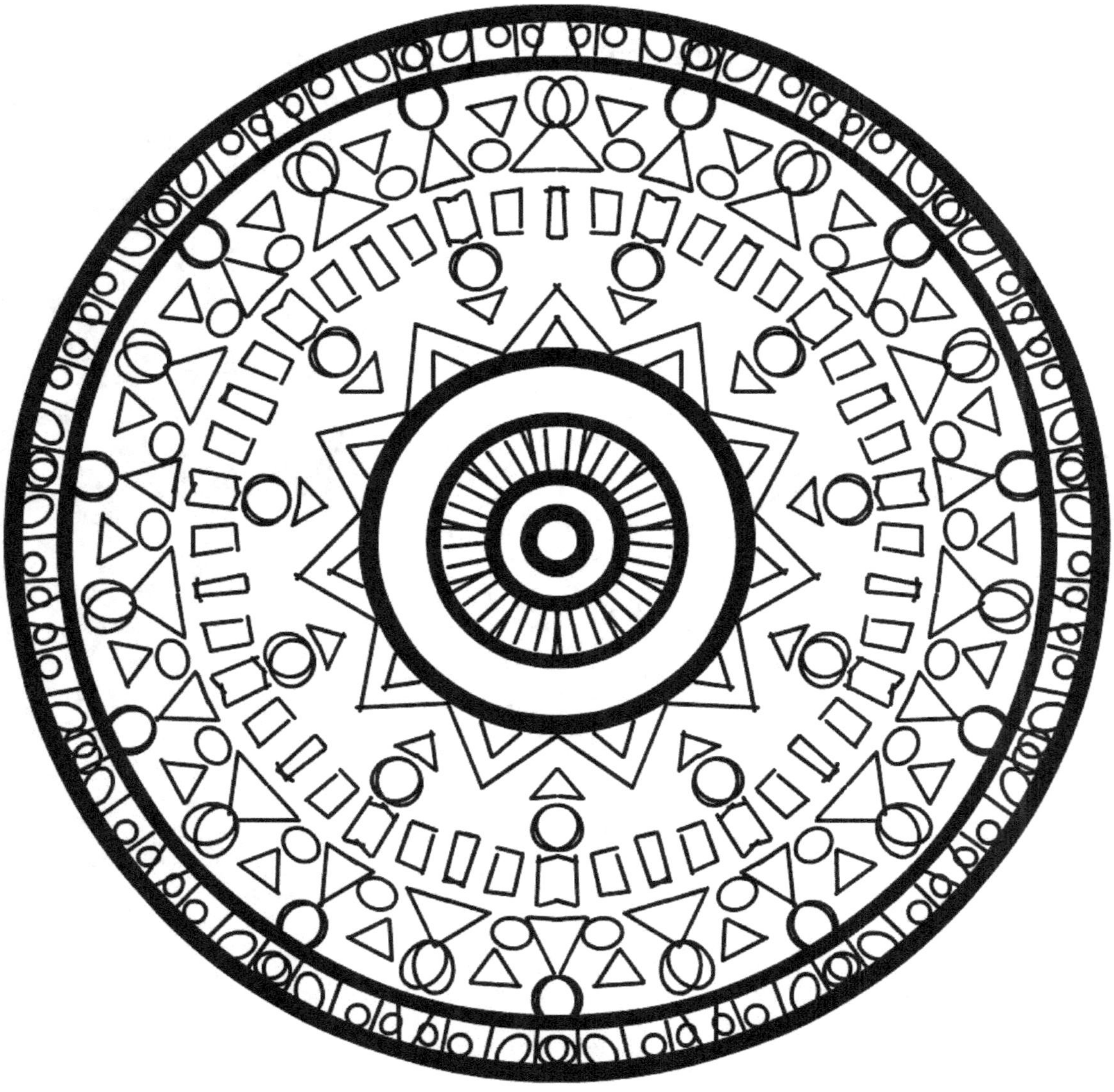

Day Twenty-two ______

5:00 ______

6:00 ______

7:00 ______

8:00 ______

9:00 ______

10:00 ______

11:00 ______

Noon ______

1:00 ______

2:00 ______

3:00 ______

4:00 ______

5:00 ______

6:00 ______

7:00 ______

8:00 ______

9:00 ______

10:00 ______

11:00 ______

Midnight ______

top priorities for today

______

______

______

______

______

Today's victories

List 5 ways to be thoughtful.

______

______

______

______

______

______

______

______

BE THOUGHTFUL

The Stella Society Workout

Exercise	Set 1	Set 2	Set 3	Set 4	Set 5	notes

Time started: ____________ Time ended: _____________

Location: ____

Feelings before training:

Feelings after training

NUTRITION

Meal 1

time eaten: _________

Meal 2

time eaten: _________

Meal 3

time eaten: _________

Meal 4

time eaten: _________

Meal 5

time eaten: _________

Hydration

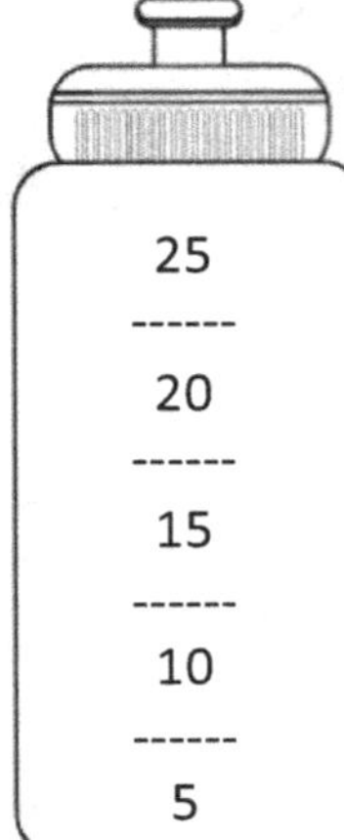

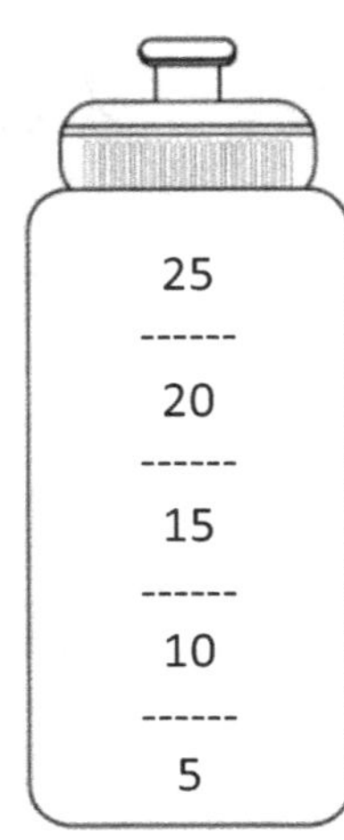

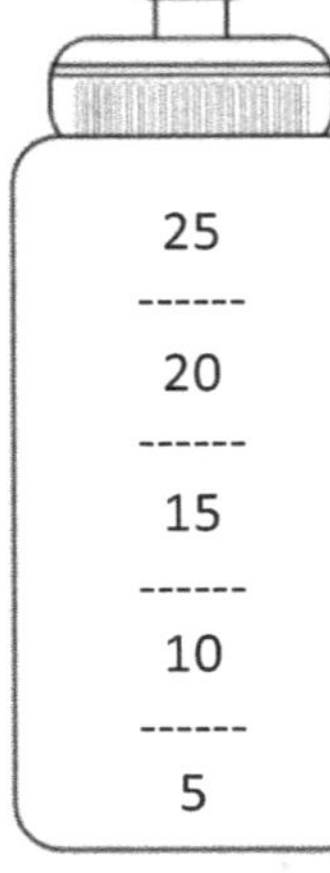

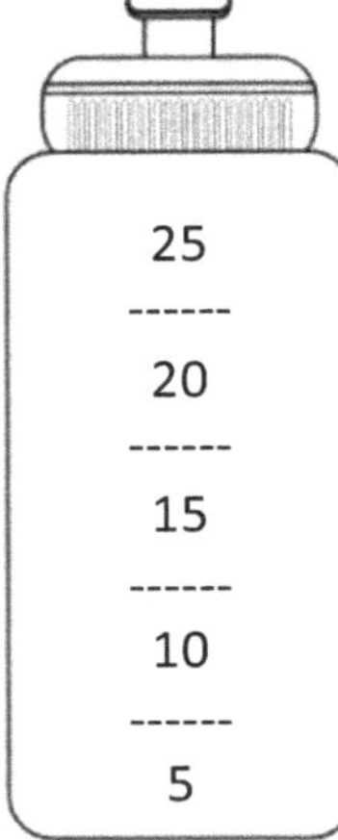

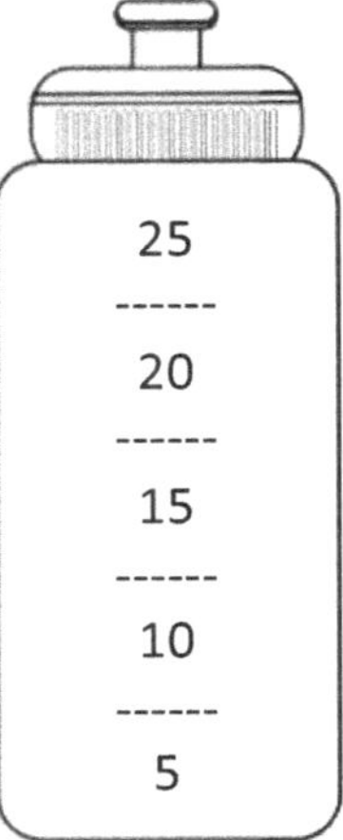

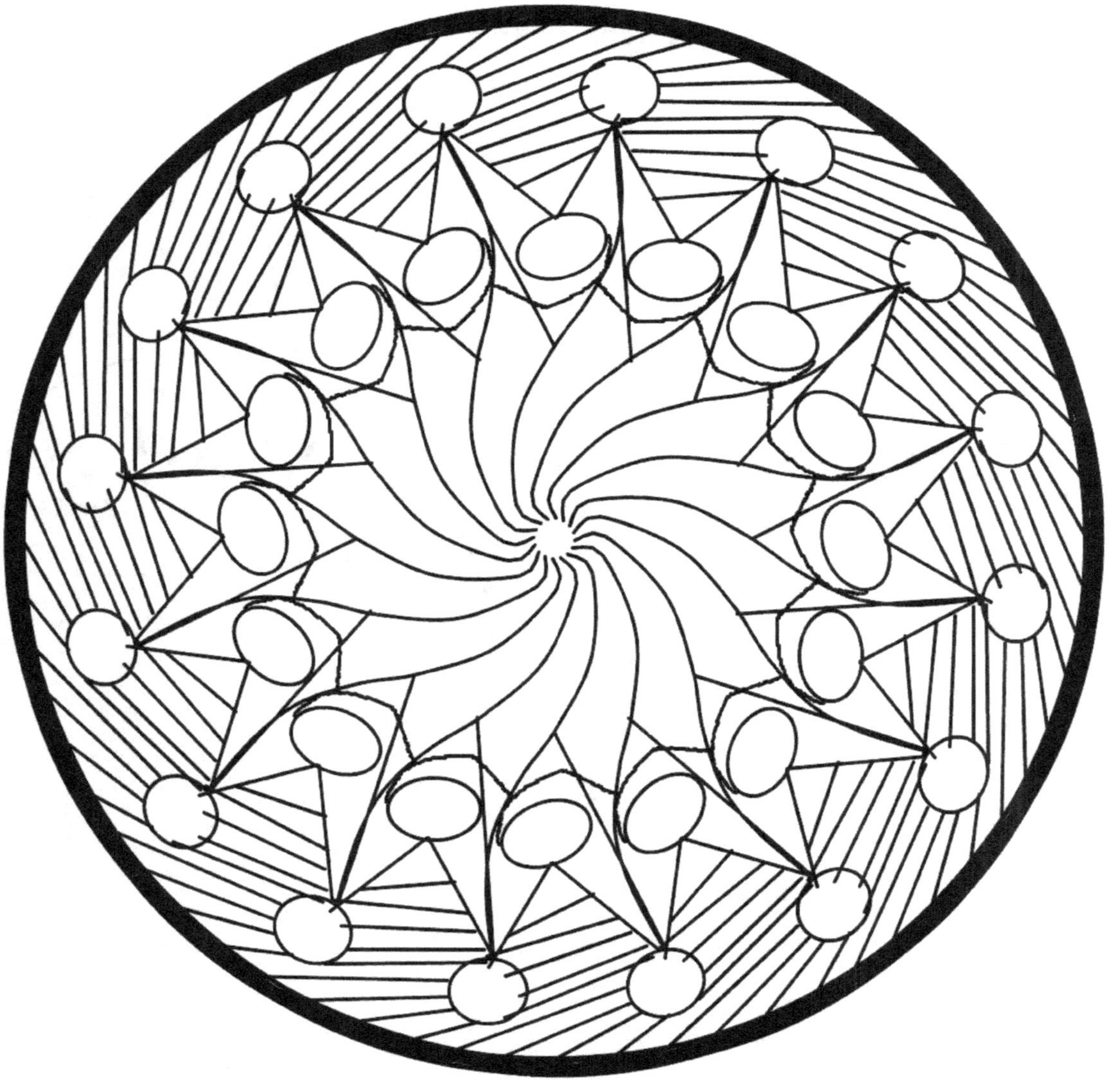

Day Twenty-three ______

5:00 ______
6:00 ______
7:00 ______
8:00 ______
9:00 ______
10:00 ______
11:00 ______
Noon ______
1:00 ______
2:00 ______
3:00 ______
4:00 ______
5:00 ______
6:00 ______
7:00 ______
8:00 ______
9:00 ______
10:00 ______
11:00 ______
Midnight ______

top priorities for today

Today's victories

Why should you be unapologetic?

The Stella Society Workout

Exercise	Set 1	Set 2	Set 3	Set 4	Set 5	notes

Time started: ____________ Time ended: _____________

Location: ____

Feelings before training:

Feelings after training

NUTRITION

Meal 1

time eaten: _________

Meal 2

time eaten: _________

Meal 3

time eaten: _________

Meal 4

time eaten: _________

Meal 5

time eaten: _________

Hydration

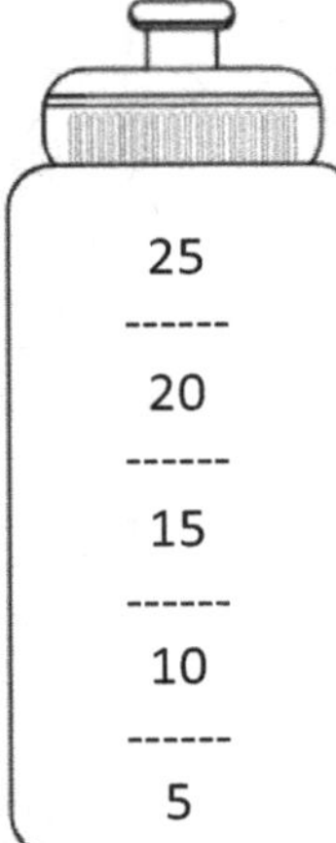

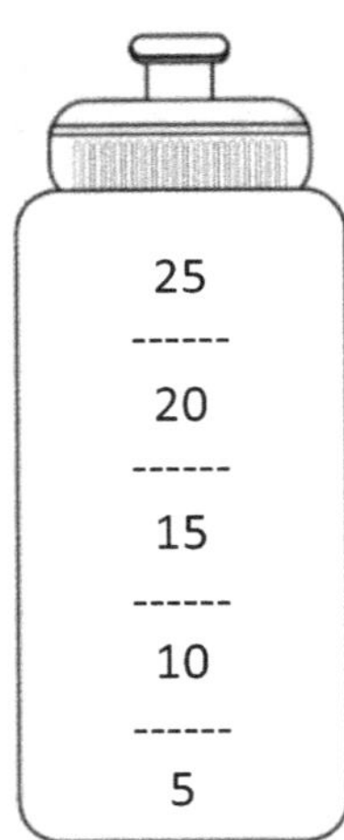

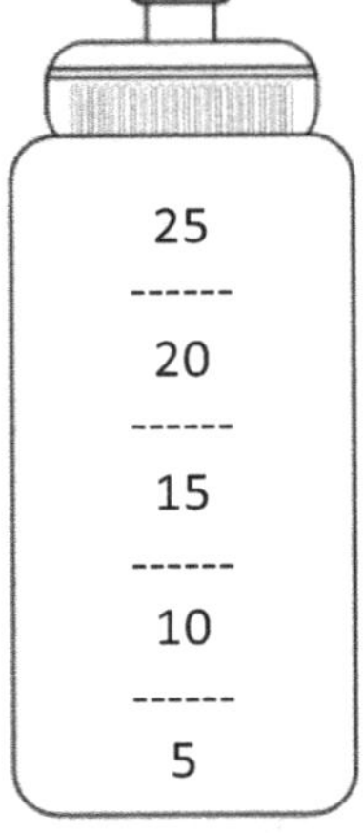

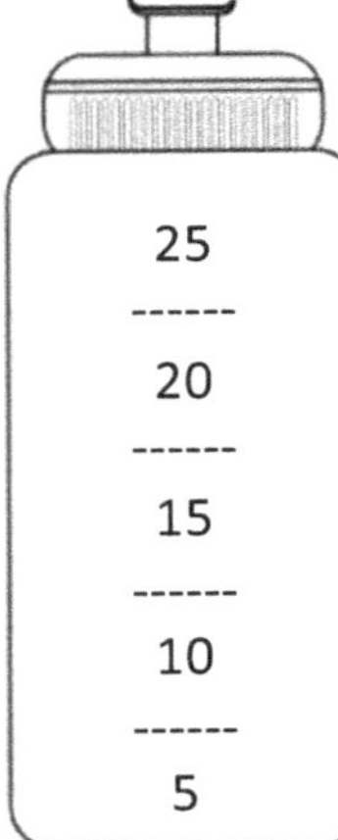

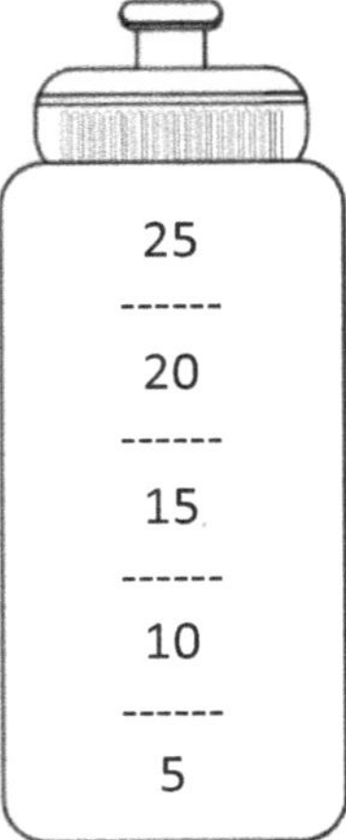

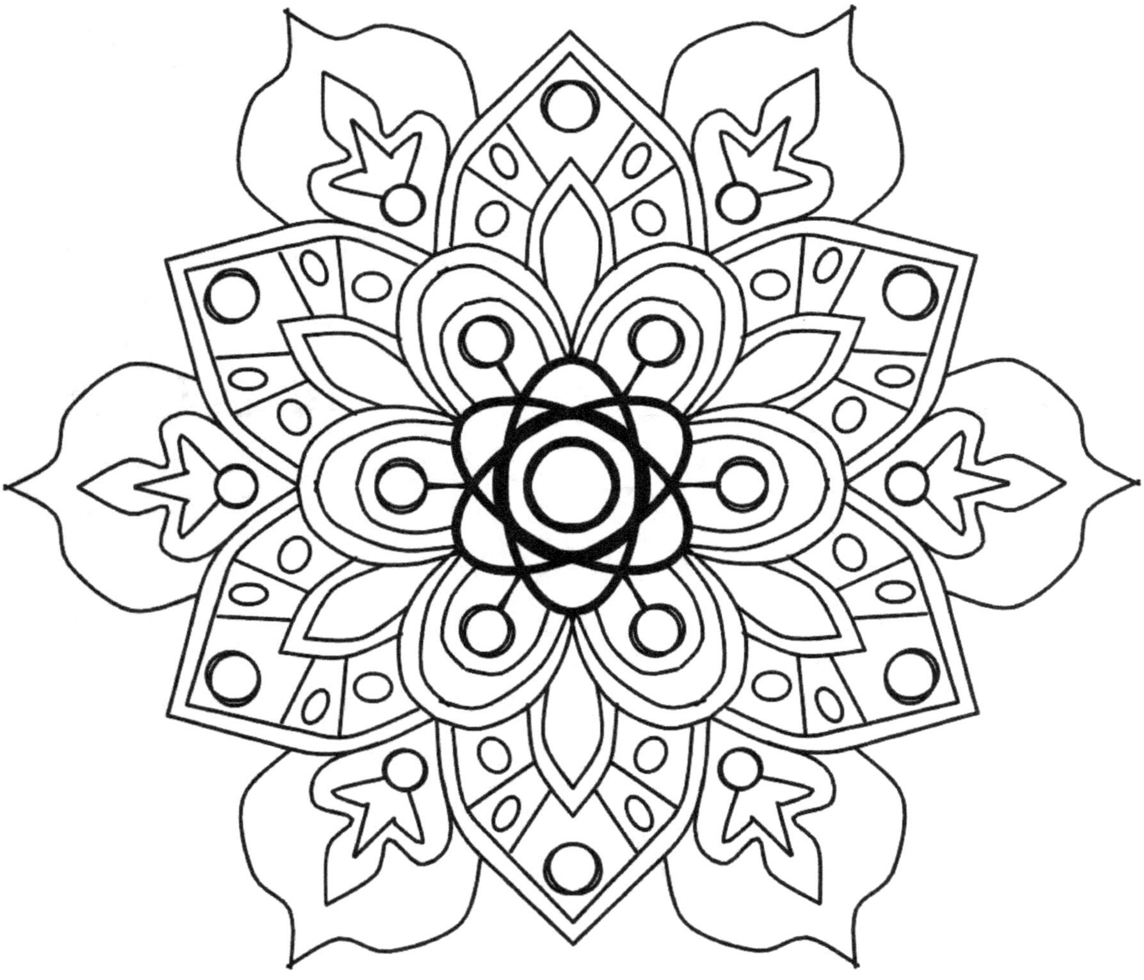

Day Twenty-four ______

5:00 ______
6:00 ______
7:00 ______
8:00 ______
9:00 ______
10:00 ______
11:00 ______
Noon ______
1:00 ______
2:00 ______
3:00 ______
4:00 ______
5:00 ______
6:00 ______
7:00 ______
8:00 ______
9:00 ______
10:00 ______
11:00 ______
Midnight ______

top priorities for today

______
______
______
______
______

Today's victories

What can you set on fire with your fierceness?

______
______
______
______
______
______
______
______

The Stella Society Workout

Exercise	Set 1	Set 2	Set 3	Set 4	Set 5	notes

Time started: _____________ Time ended: ______________

Location: ____

Feelings before training:

Feelings after training

NUTRITION

Meal 1

time eaten: _________

Meal 2

time eaten: _________

Meal 3

time eaten: _________

Meal 4

time eaten: _________

Meal 5

time eaten: _________

Hydration

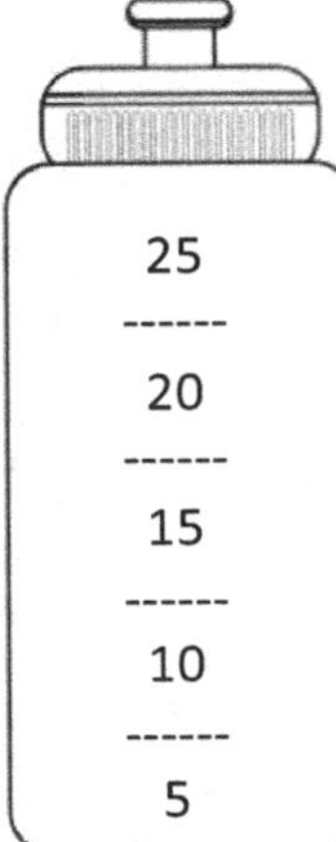

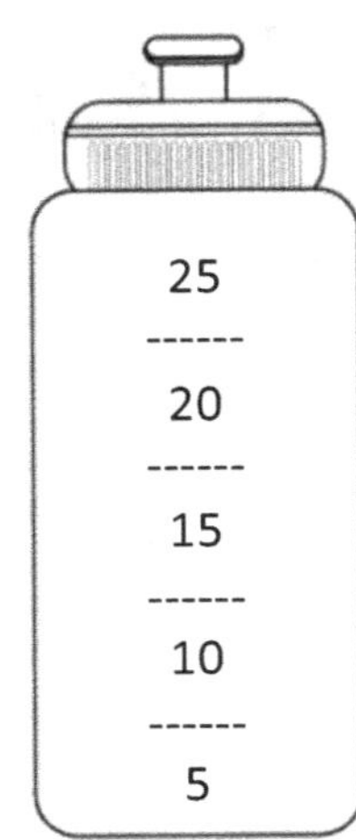

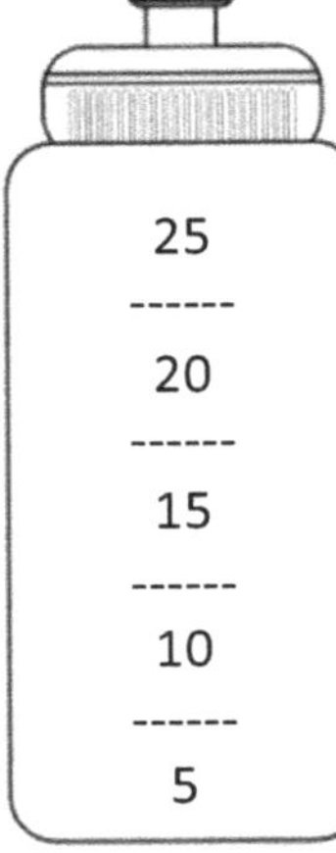

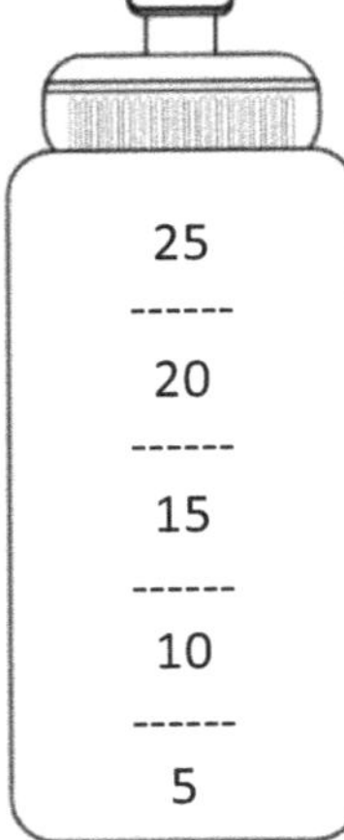

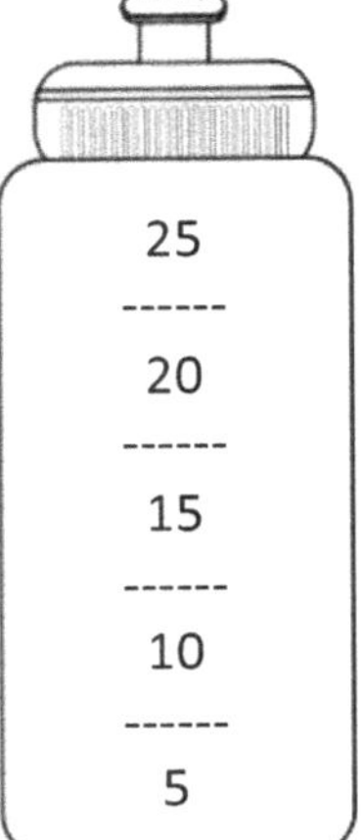

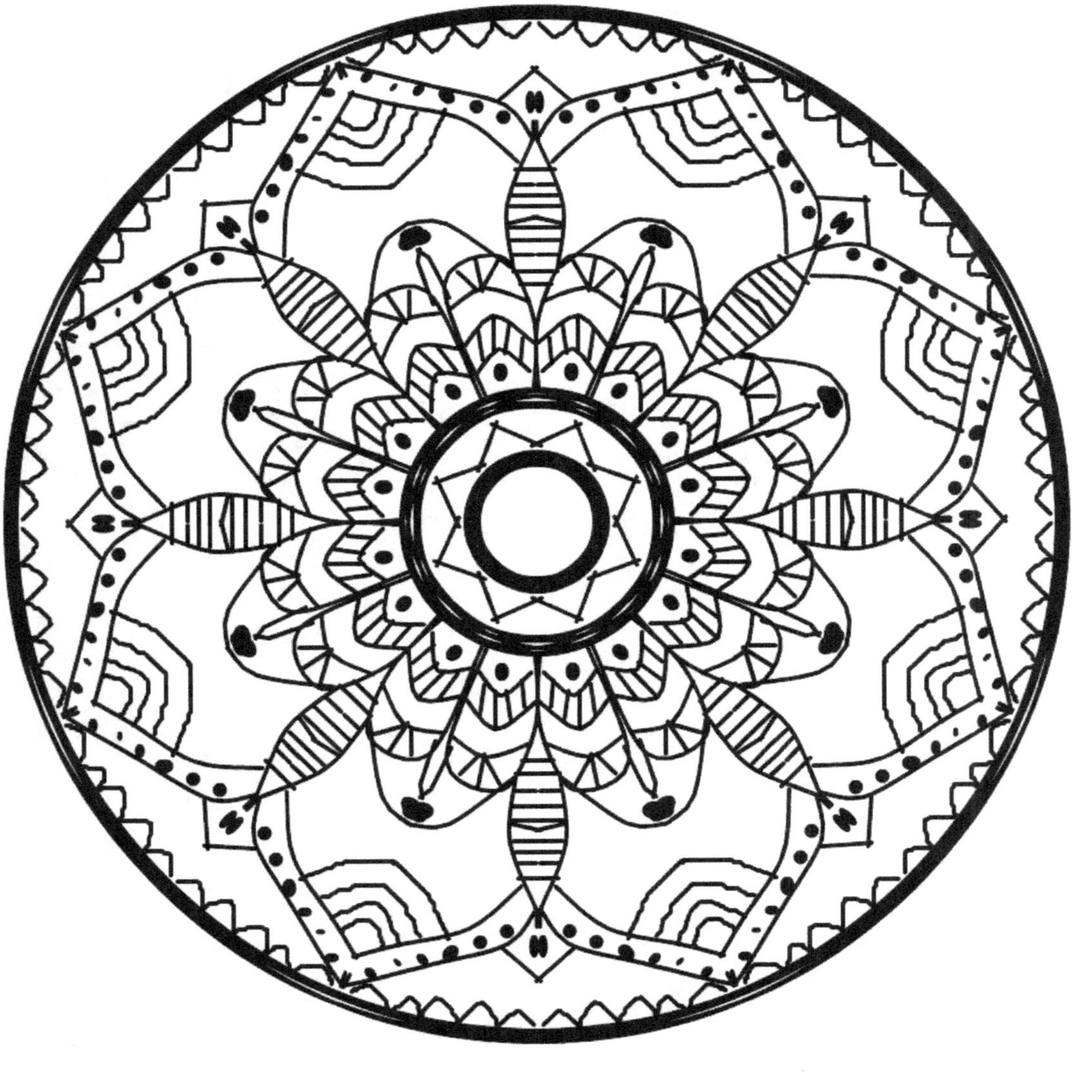

Day Twenty-five ______

5:00 ____________________

6:00 ____________________

7:00 ____________________

8:00 ____________________

9:00 ____________________

10:00 ____________________

11:00 ____________________

Noon ____________________

1:00 ____________________

2:00 ____________________

3:00 ____________________

4:00 ____________________

5:00 ____________________

6:00 ____________________

7:00 ____________________

8:00 ____________________

9:00 ____________________

10:00 ____________________

11:00 ____________________

Midnight ____________________

top priorities for today

Today's victories

Make it your mission to stay positive. Write your positive mission statement.

BE POSITIVE

The Stella Society Workout

Exercise	Set 1	Set 2	Set 3	Set 4	Set 5	notes

Time started: ____________ Time ended: _____________

Location: ____

Feelings before training:

Feelings after training

NUTRITION

Meal 1

time eaten: _________

Meal 2

time eaten: _________

Meal 3

time eaten: _________

Meal 4

time eaten: _________

Meal 5

time eaten: _________

Hydration

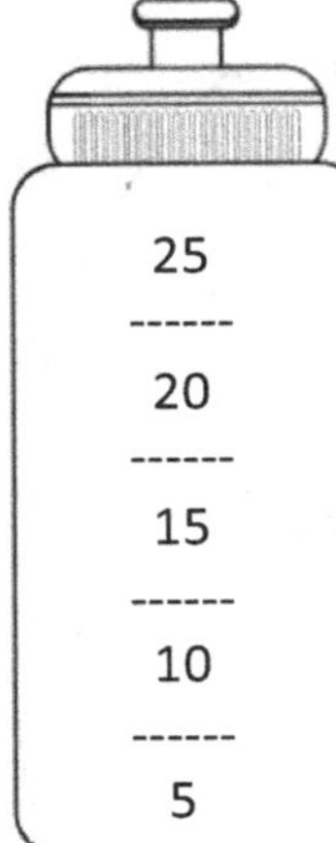

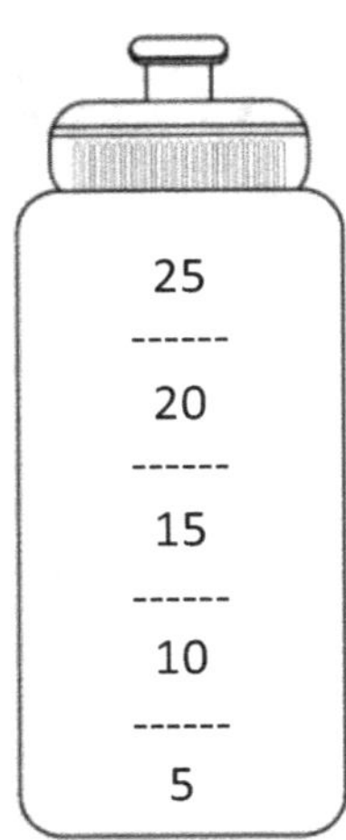

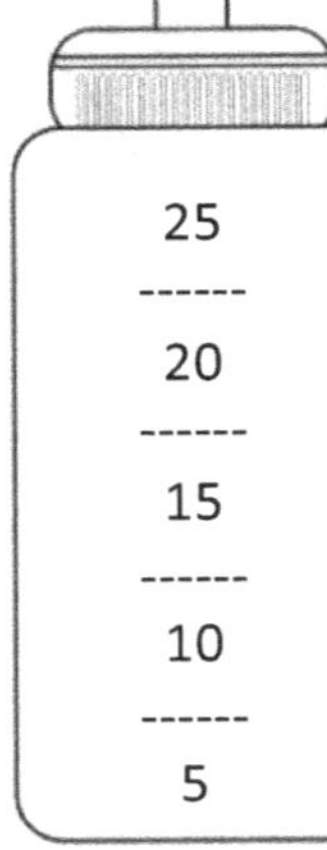

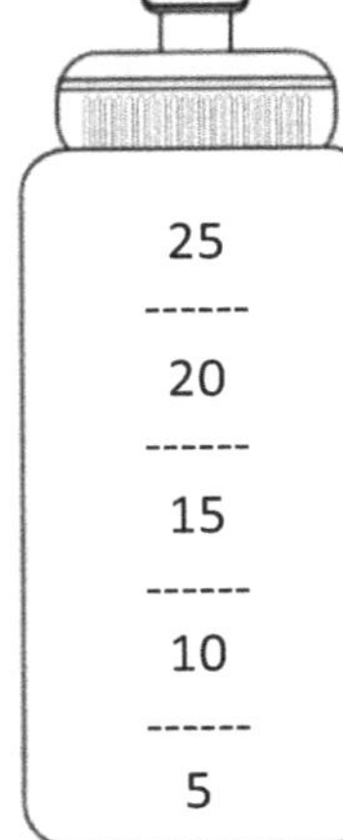

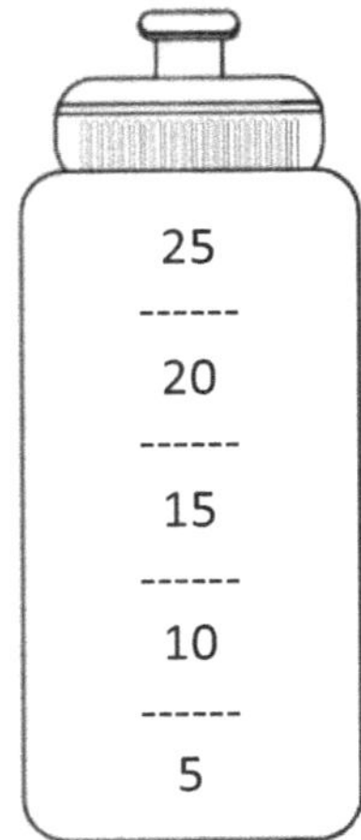

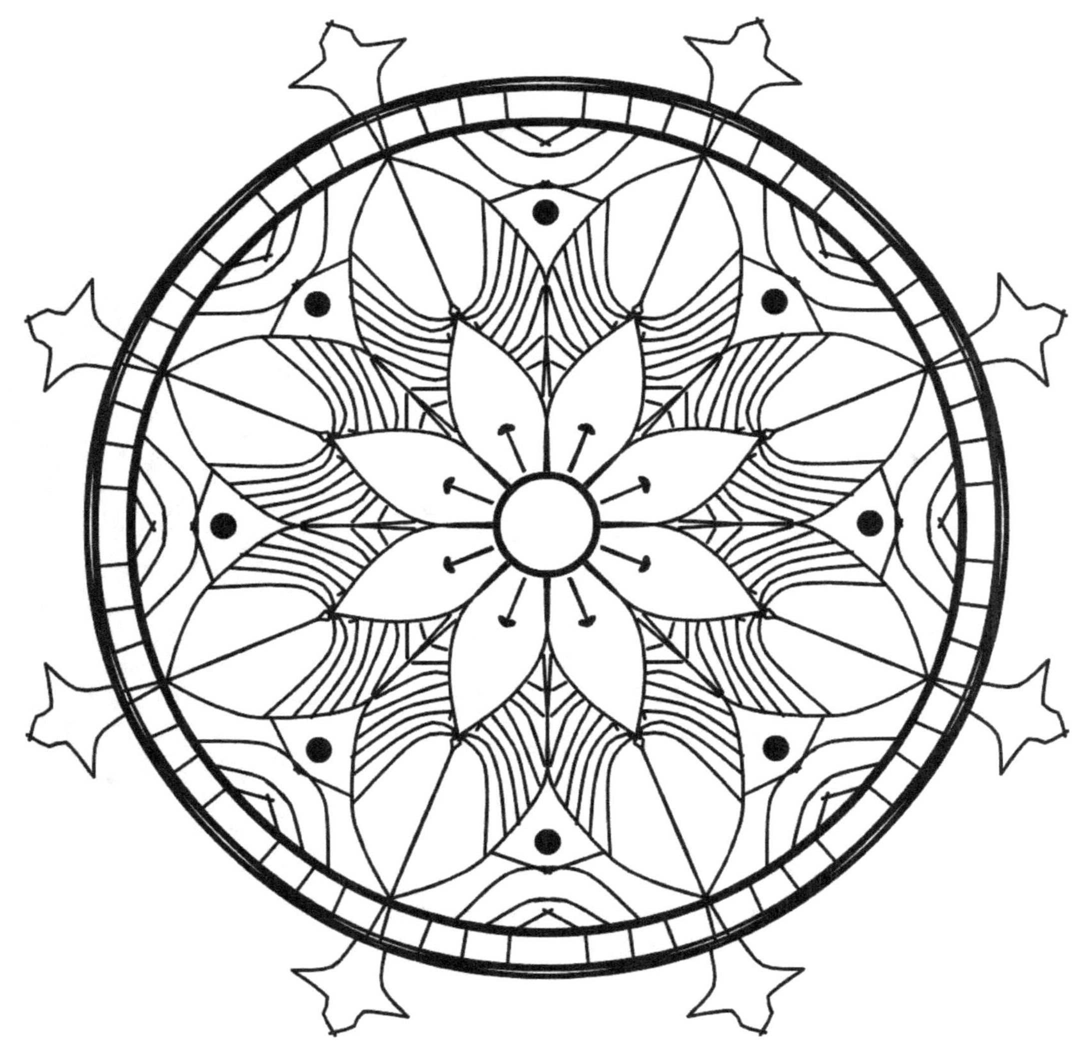

Day Twenty-six ______

5:00 ______

6:00 ______

7:00 ______

8:00 ______

9:00 ______

10:00 ______

11:00 ______

Noon ______

1:00 ______

2:00 ______

3:00 ______

4:00 ______

5:00 ______

6:00 ______

7:00 ______

8:00 ______

9:00 ______

10:00 ______

11:00 ______

Midnight ______

top priorities for today

______

______

______

______

______

Today's victories

What give you your inner energy?

______

______

______

______

______

______

______

______

The Stella Society Workout

Exercise	Set 1	Set 2	Set 3	Set 4	Set 5	notes

Time started: ____________ Time ended: _____________

Location: ____

Feelings before training:

Feelings after training

NUTRITION

Meal 1

time eaten: _________

Meal 2

time eaten: _________

Meal 3

time eaten: _________

Meal 4

time eaten: _________

Meal 5

time eaten: _________

Hydration

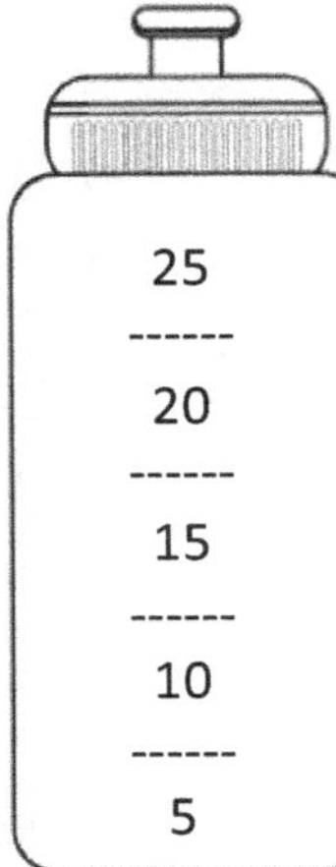

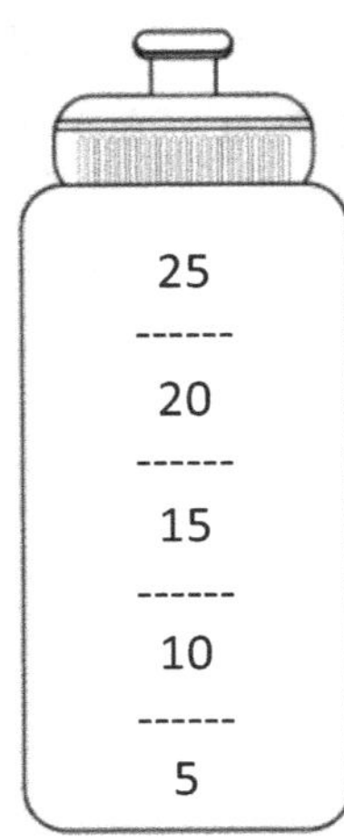

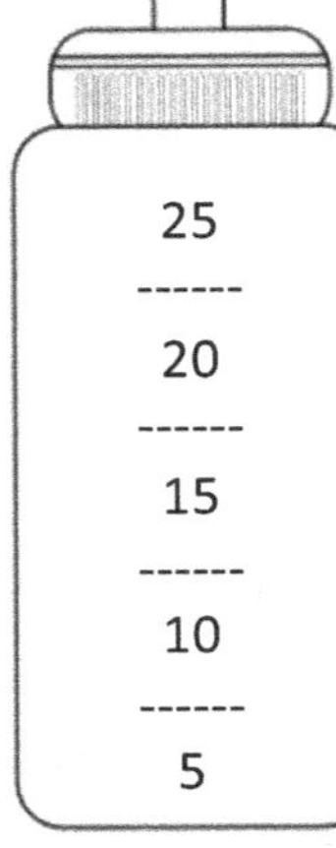

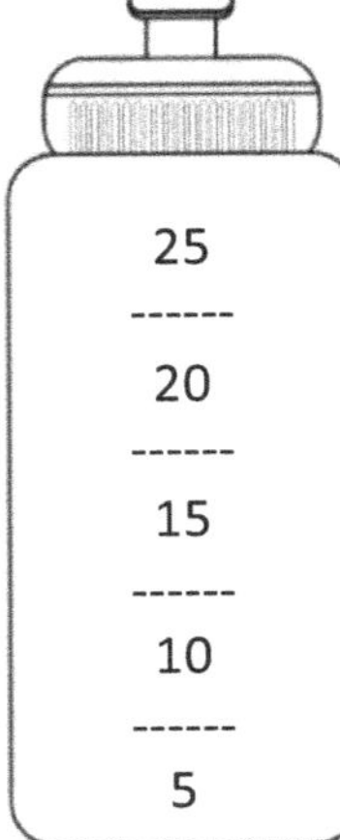

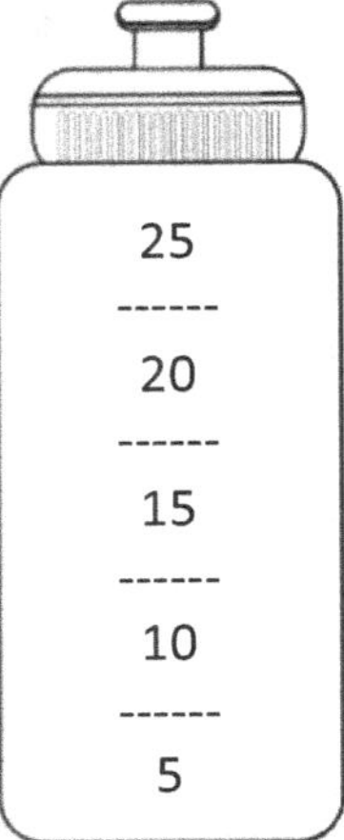

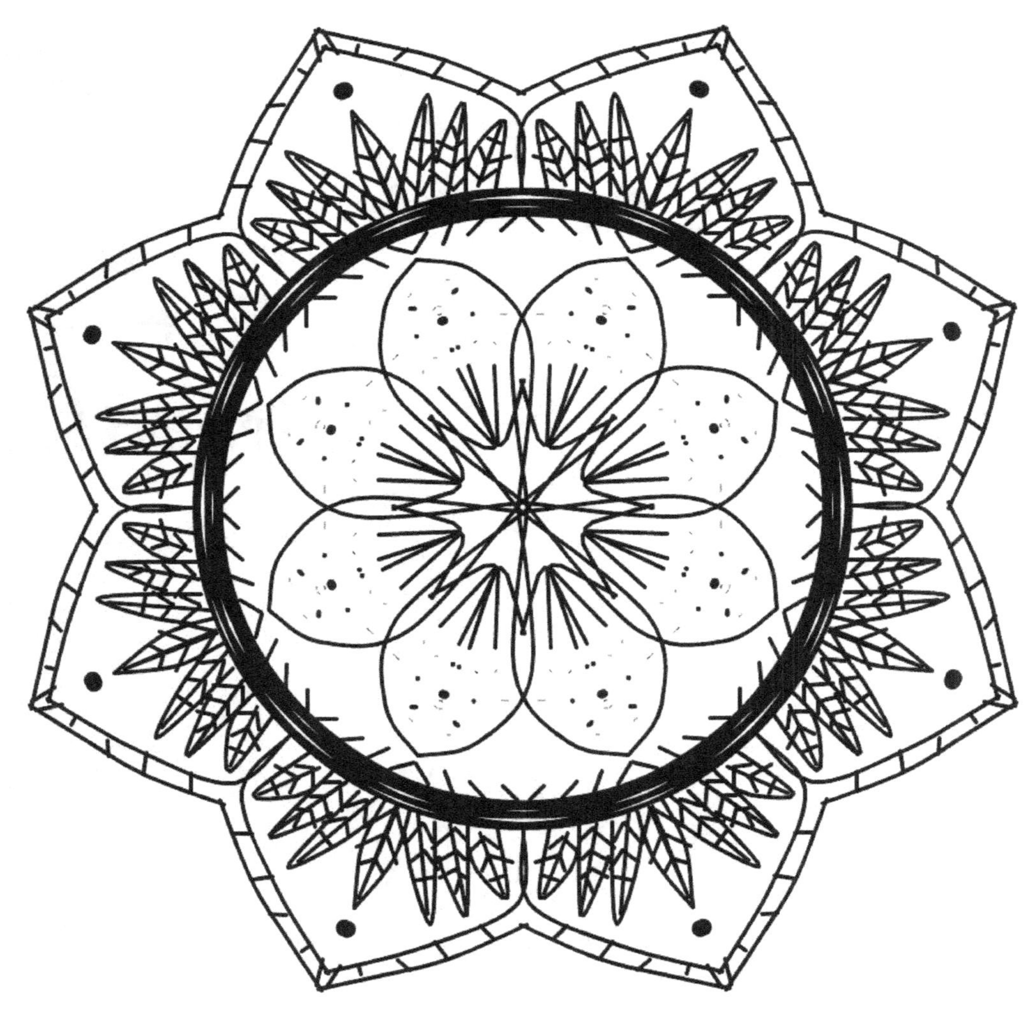

Day Twenty-seven ______

5:00 ______
6:00 ______
7:00 ______
8:00 ______
9:00 ______
10:00 ______
11:00 ______
Noon ______
1:00 ______
2:00 ______
3:00 ______
4:00 ______
5:00 ______
6:00 ______
7:00 ______
8:00 ______
9:00 ______
10:00 ______
11:00 ______
Midnight ______

top priorities for today

______
______
______
______
______

Today's victories

What have you stopped, but won't stop again?

______
______
______
______
______
______
______
______

The Stella Society Workout

Exercise	Set 1	Set 2	Set 3	Set 4	Set 5	notes

Time started: ______________ Time ended: _______________

Location: ____

Feelings before training:

Feelings after training

NUTRITION

Meal 1

time eaten: _________

Meal 2

time eaten: _________

Meal 3

time eaten: _________

Meal 4

time eaten: _________

Meal 5

time eaten: _________

Hydration

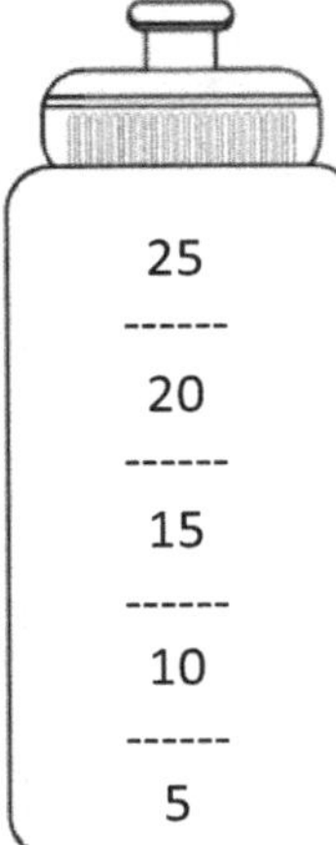

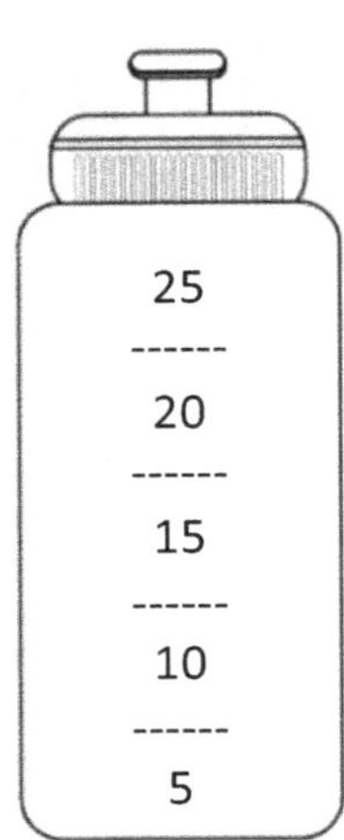

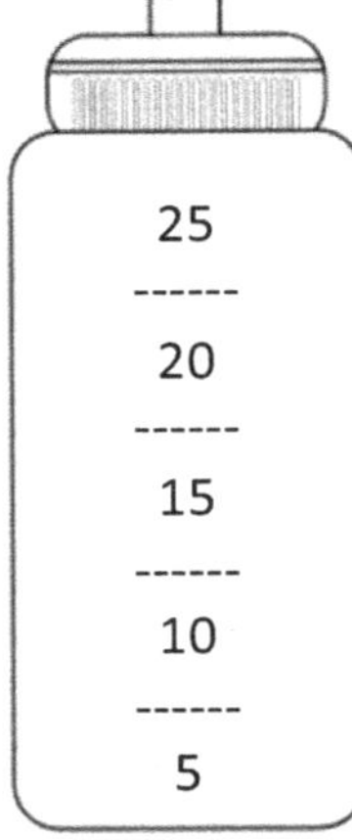

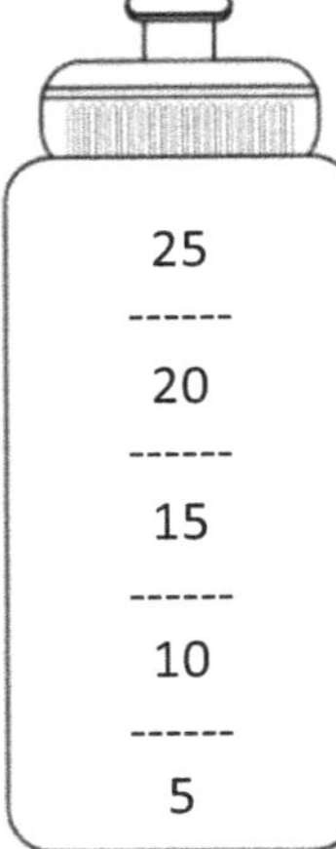

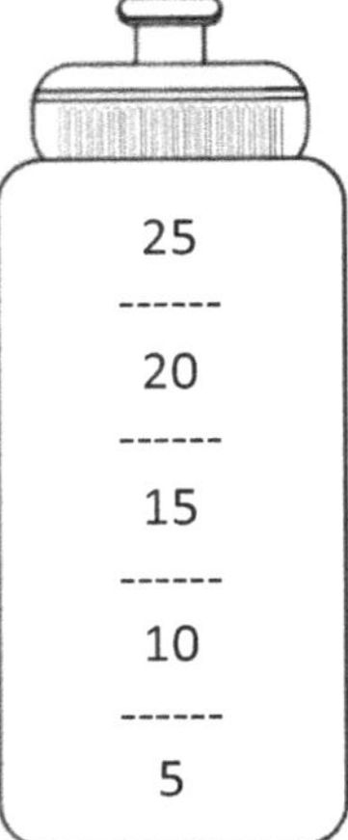

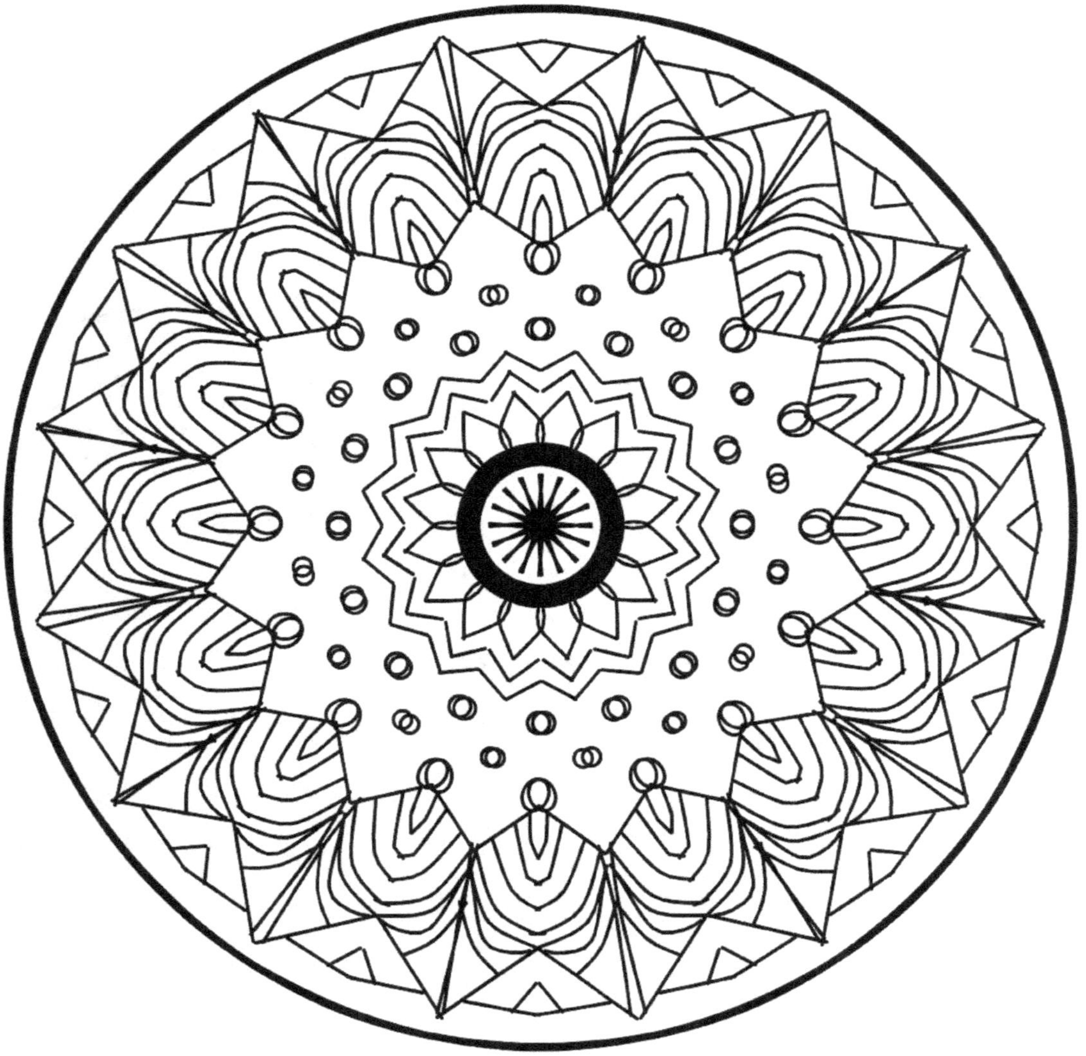

Day Twenty-eight ______

5:00 ______
6:00 ______
7:00 ______
8:00 ______
9:00 ______
10:00 ______
11:00 ______
Noon ______
1:00 ______
2:00 ______
3:00 ______
4:00 ______
5:00 ______
6:00 ______
7:00 ______
8:00 ______
9:00 ______
10:00 ______
11:00 ______
Midnight ______

top priorities for today

______
______
______
______
______

Today's victories

How do identify with being a unicorn?

______
______
______
______
______
______
______
______

The Stella Society Workout

Exercise	Set 1	Set 2	Set 3	Set 4	Set 5	notes

Time started: ____________ Time ended: _____________

Location: ____

Feelings before training:

Feelings after training

NUTRITION

Meal 1

time eaten: _________

Meal 2

time eaten: _________

Meal 3

time eaten: _________

Meal 4

time eaten: _________

Meal 5

time eaten: _________

Hydration

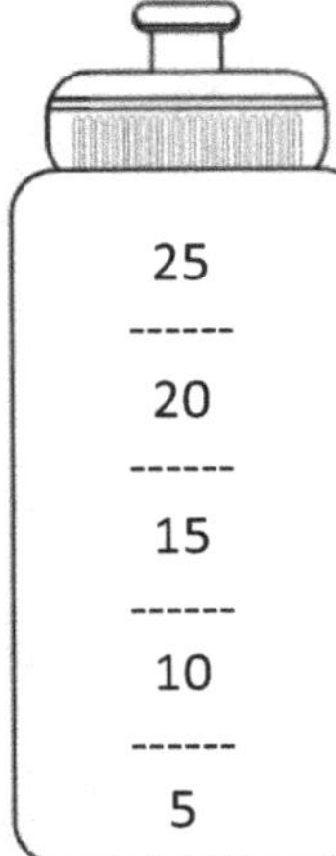

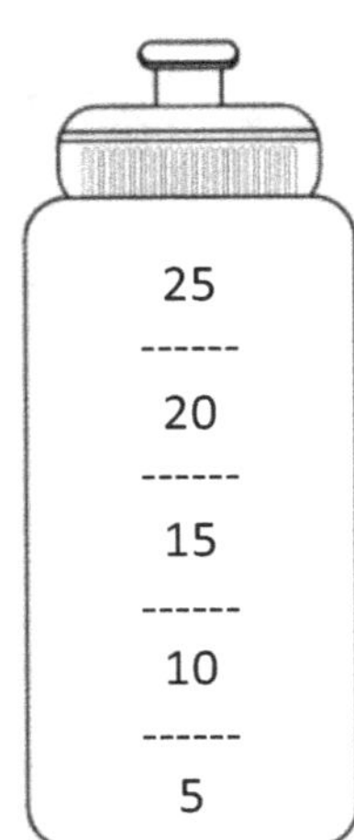

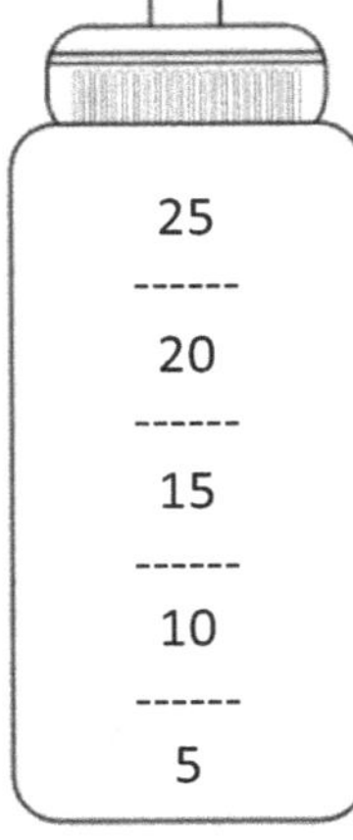

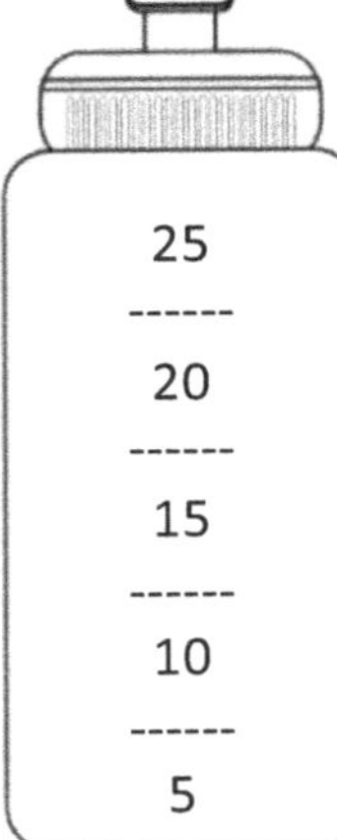

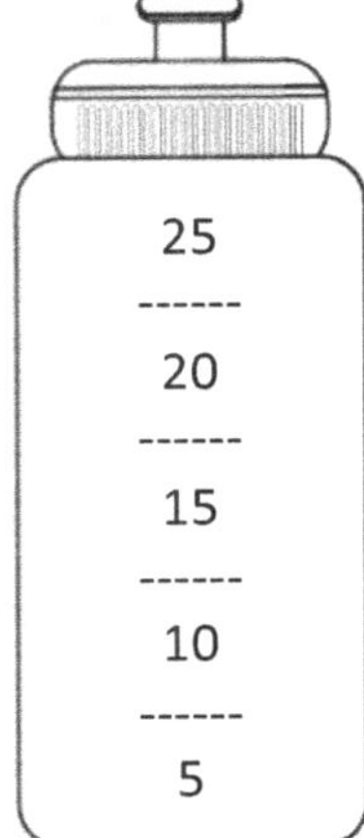

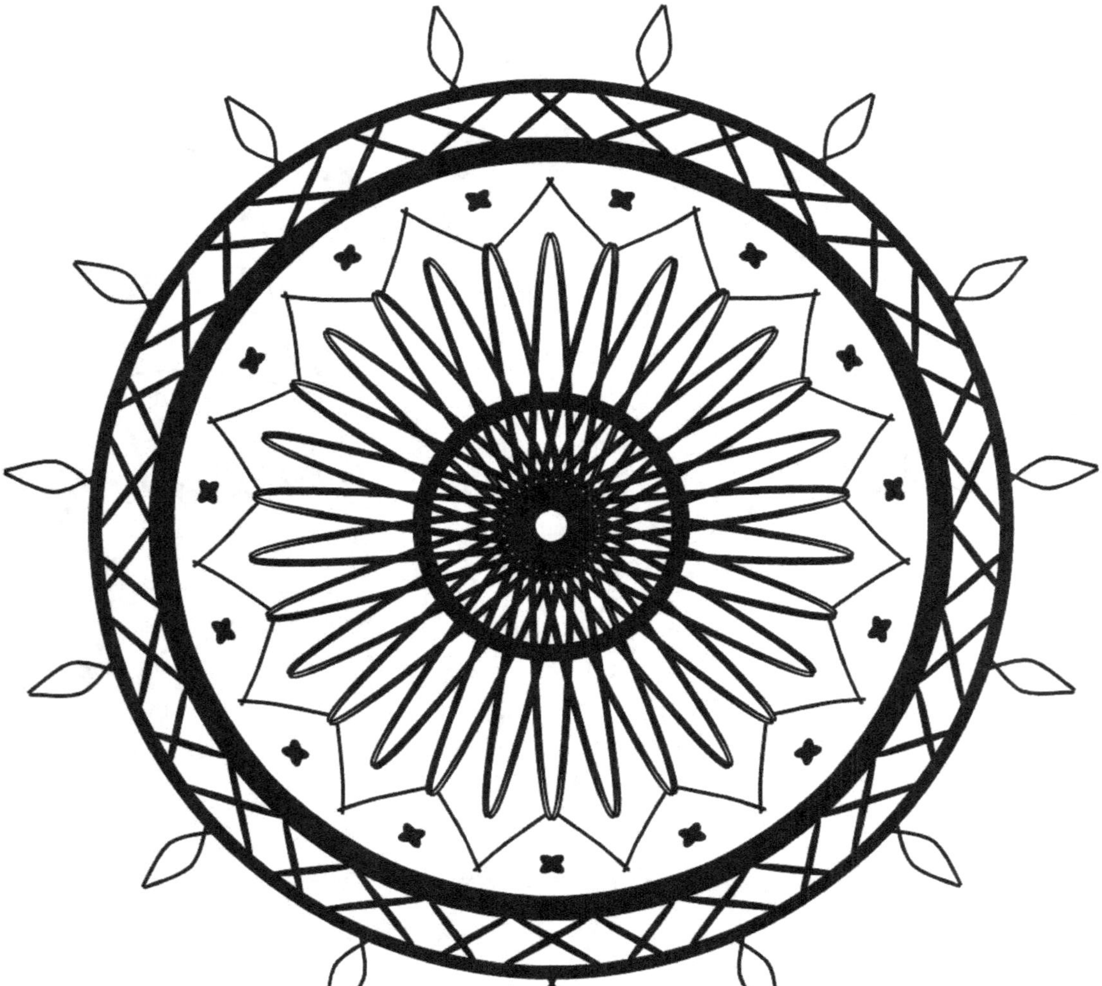

Day Twenty-nine ______

5:00 ______
6:00 ______
7:00 ______
8:00 ______
9:00 ______
10:00 ______
11:00 ______
Noon ______
1:00 ______
2:00 ______
3:00 ______
4:00 ______
5:00 ______
6:00 ______
7:00 ______
8:00 ______
9:00 ______
10:00 ______
11:00 ______
Midnight ______

top priorities for today

______
______
______
______
______

Today's victories

You have permission to be a savage. What do you do with it?

______
______
______
______
______
______
______
______

The Stella Society Workout

Exercise	Set 1	Set 2	Set 3	Set 4	Set 5	notes

Time started: ____________ Time ended: _____________

Location: ____

Feelings before training: 😊 😑 ☹️ 😝 😠 😕 😇 😎

Feelings after training 😊 😑 ☹️ 😝 😠 😕 😇 😎

NUTRITION

Meal 1

time eaten: _________

Meal 2

time eaten: _________

Meal 3

time eaten: _________

Meal 4

time eaten: _________

Meal 5

time eaten: _________

Hydration

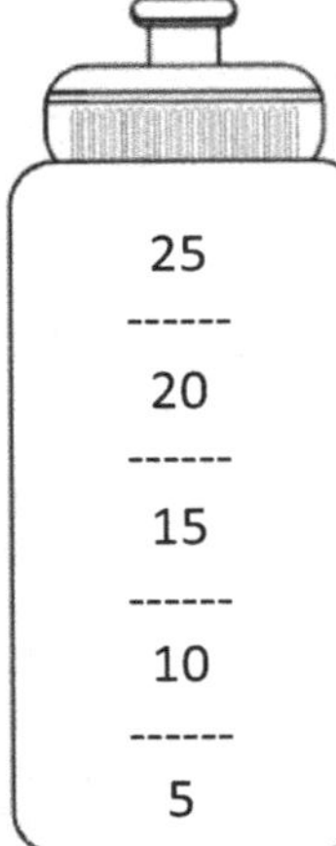

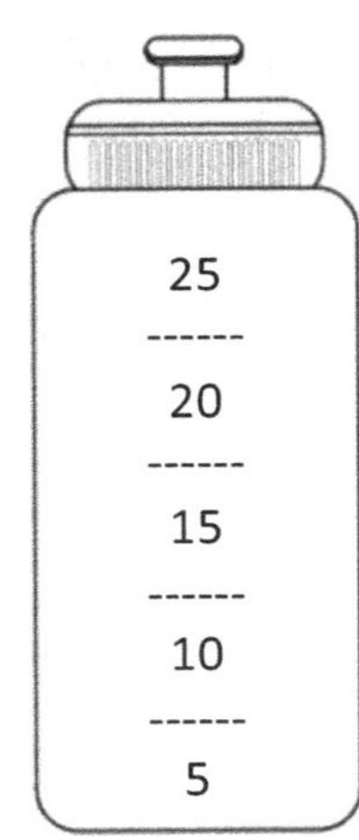

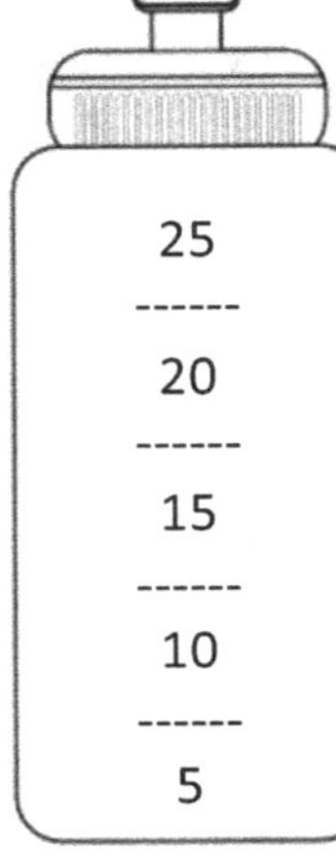

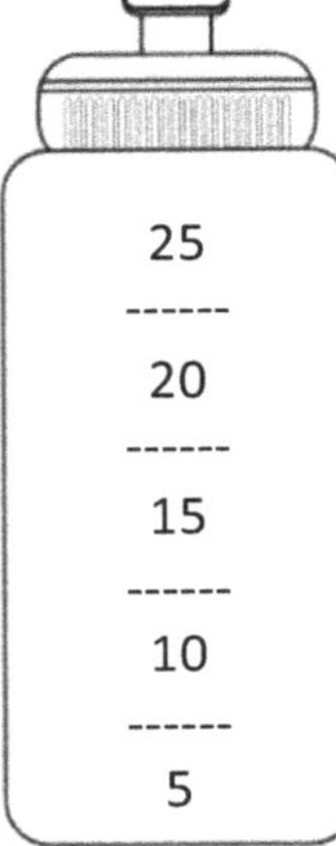

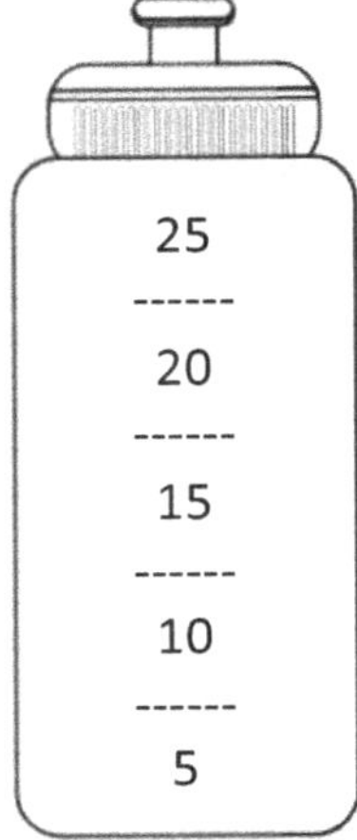

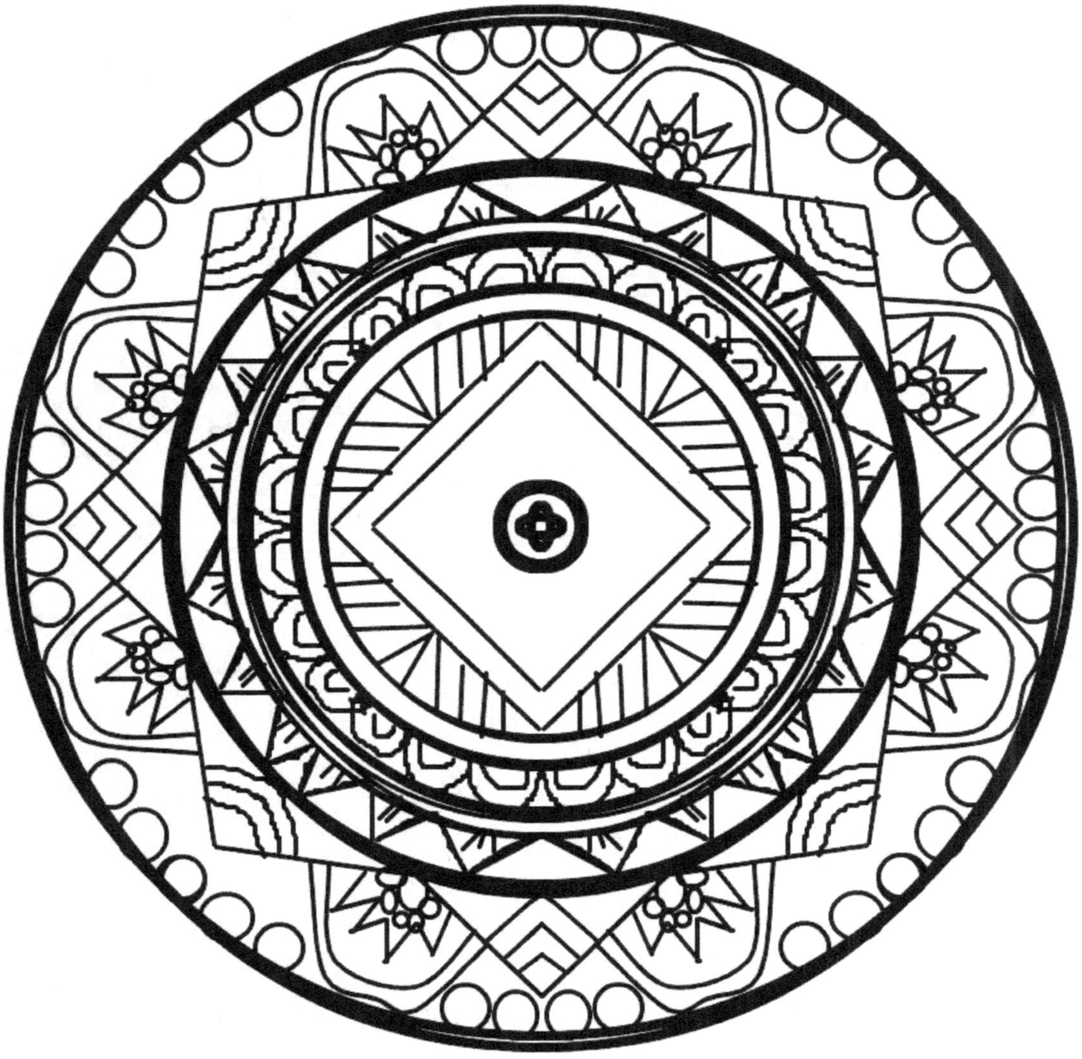

Measurements

PROGRESS

DATE: __________

Weight: ______

Neck ______

Shoulders ______

Chest ______

Bicep / upper arm left _______ right ______

Forearm left _______ right ______

Waist ______

Hips ______

Thighs left _______ right ______

Calf left _______ right ______

CHECK

It's Not A Diet,
It's A Lifestyle Change

Day Thirty ______

5:00 ____________________

6:00 ____________________

7:00 ____________________

8:00 ____________________

9:00 ____________________

10:00 ____________________

11:00 ____________________

Noon ____________________

1:00 ____________________

2:00 ____________________

3:00 ____________________

4:00 ____________________

5:00 ____________________

6:00 ____________________

7:00 ____________________

8:00 ____________________

9:00 ____________________

10:00 ____________________

11:00 ____________________

Midnight ____________________

top priorities for today

____

____

____

____

____

Today's victories

How can you be powerful and sensitive at the same time?

____

____

____

____

____

____

____

____

The Stella Society Workout

Exercise	Set 1	Set 2	Set 3	Set 4	Set 5	notes

Time started: ____________ Time ended: _____________

Location: ____

Feelings before training:

Feelings after training

NUTRITION

Meal 1

time eaten: _________

Meal 2

time eaten: _________

Meal 3

time eaten: _________

Meal 4

time eaten: _________

Meal 5

time eaten: _________

Hydration

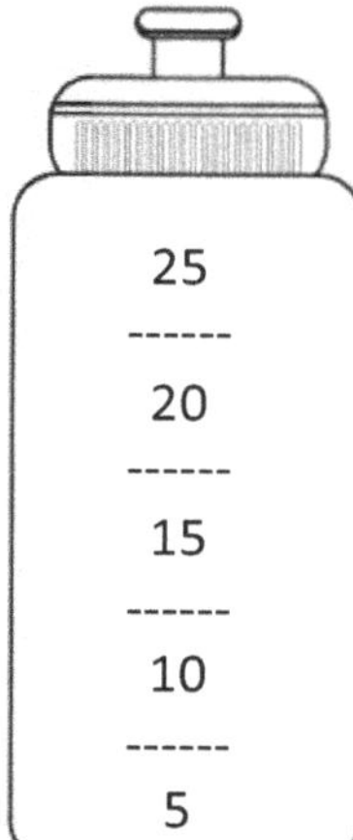

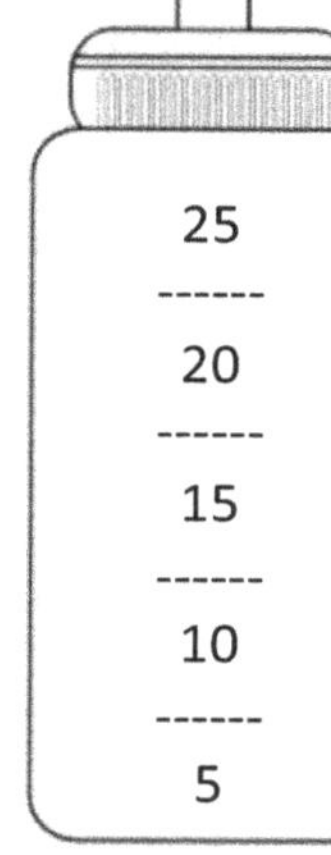

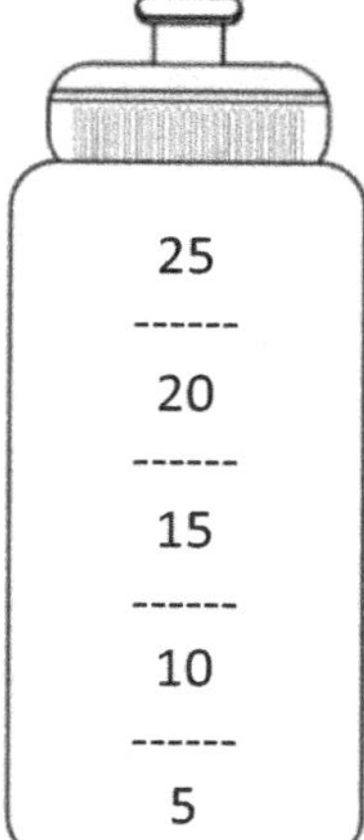

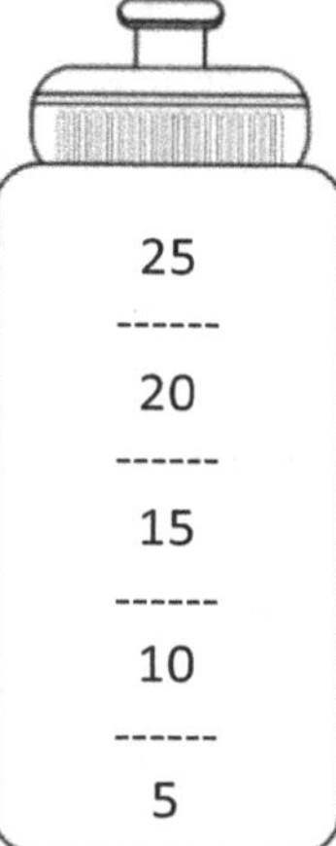

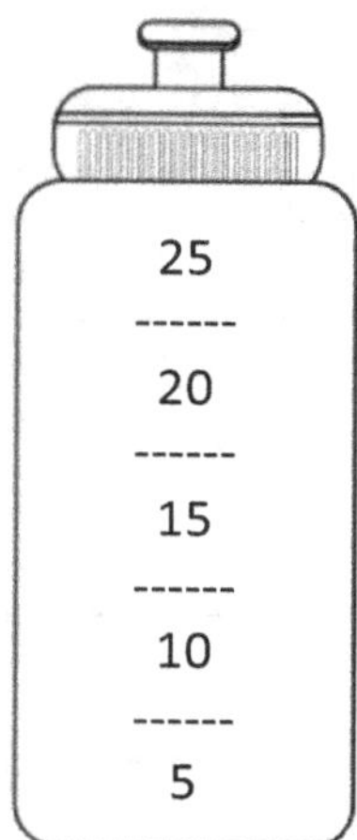

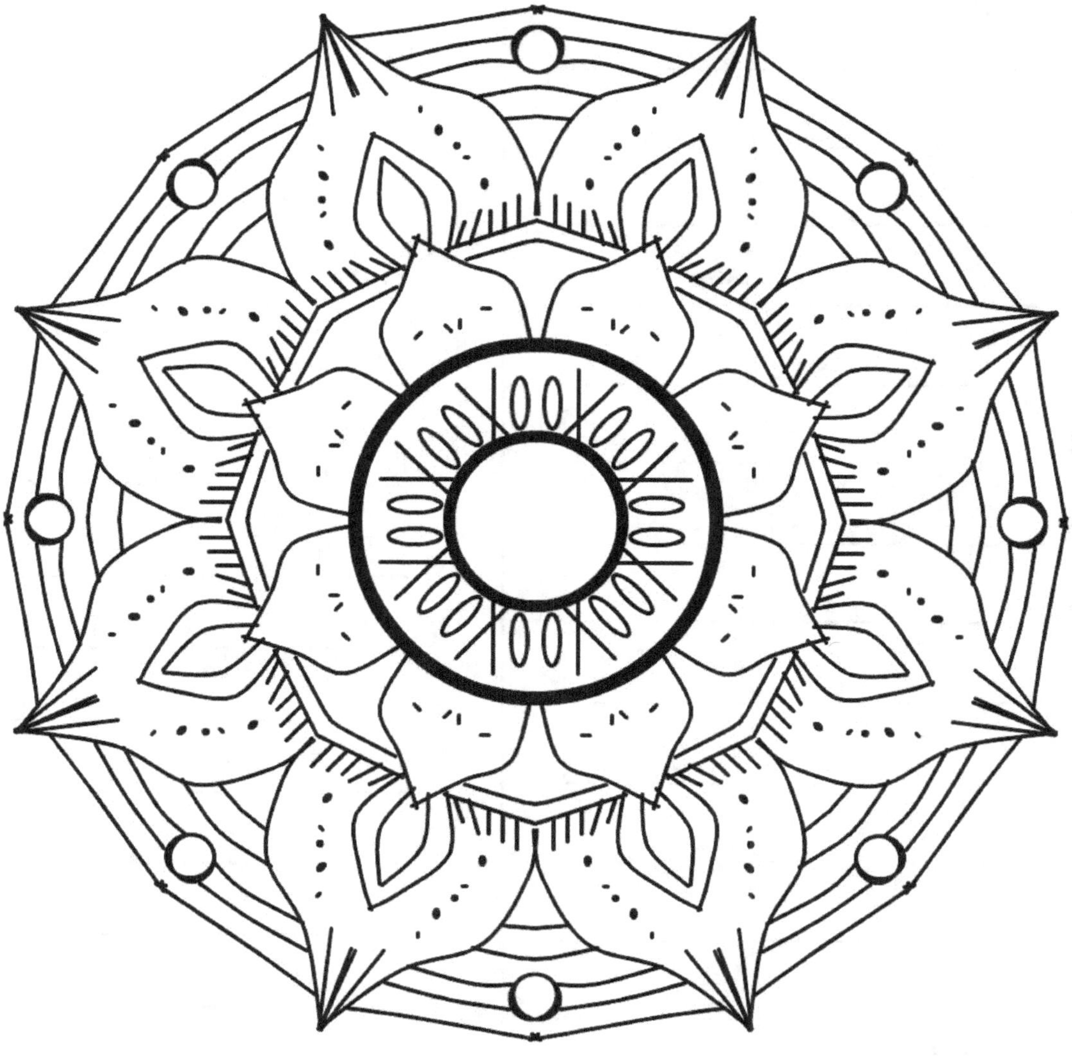

Day Thirty-one ______

5:00 ________________
6:00 ________________
7:00 ________________
8:00 ________________
9:00 ________________
10:00 ________________
11:00 ________________
Noon ________________
1:00 ________________
2:00 ________________
3:00 ________________
4:00 ________________
5:00 ________________
6:00 ________________
7:00 ________________
8:00 ________________
9:00 ________________
10:00 ________________
11:00 ________________
Midnight ________________

top priorities for today

____
____
____
____
____

Today's victories

Is being forceful a bad thing?

____
____
____
____
____
____
____
____

The Stella Society Workout

Exercise	Set 1	Set 2	Set 3	Set 4	Set 5	notes

Time started: ____________ Time ended: _____________

Location: ____

Feelings before training:

Feelings after training

NUTRITION

Meal 1

time eaten: _________

Meal 2

time eaten: _________

Meal 3

time eaten: _________

Meal 4

time eaten: _________

Meal 5

time eaten: _________

Hydration

25
20
15
10
5
25
20
15
10
5
25
20
15
10
5
25
20
15
10
5
25
20
15
10
5

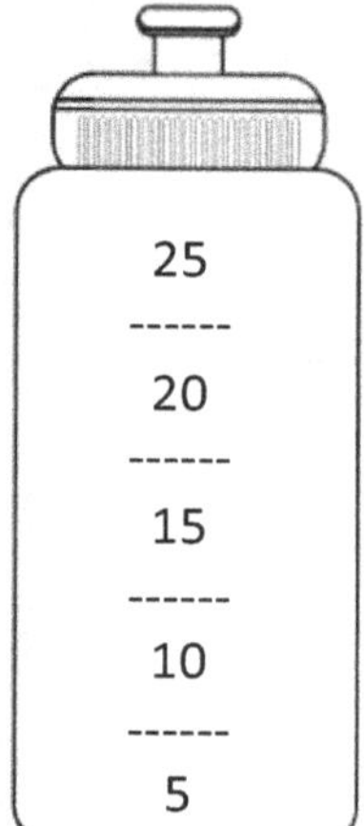

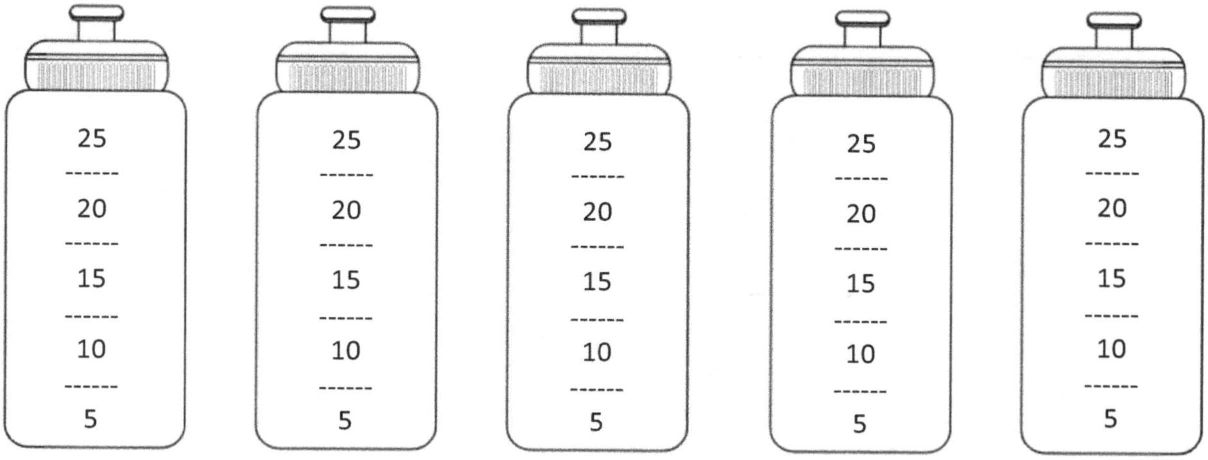

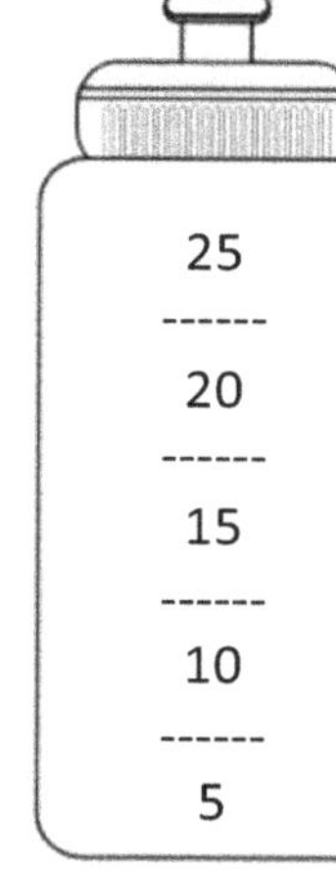

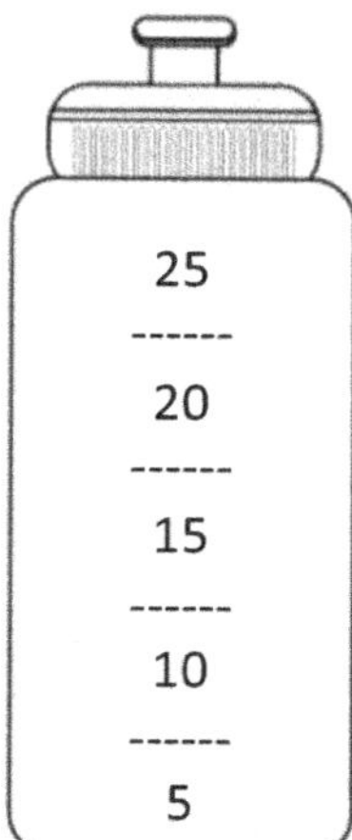

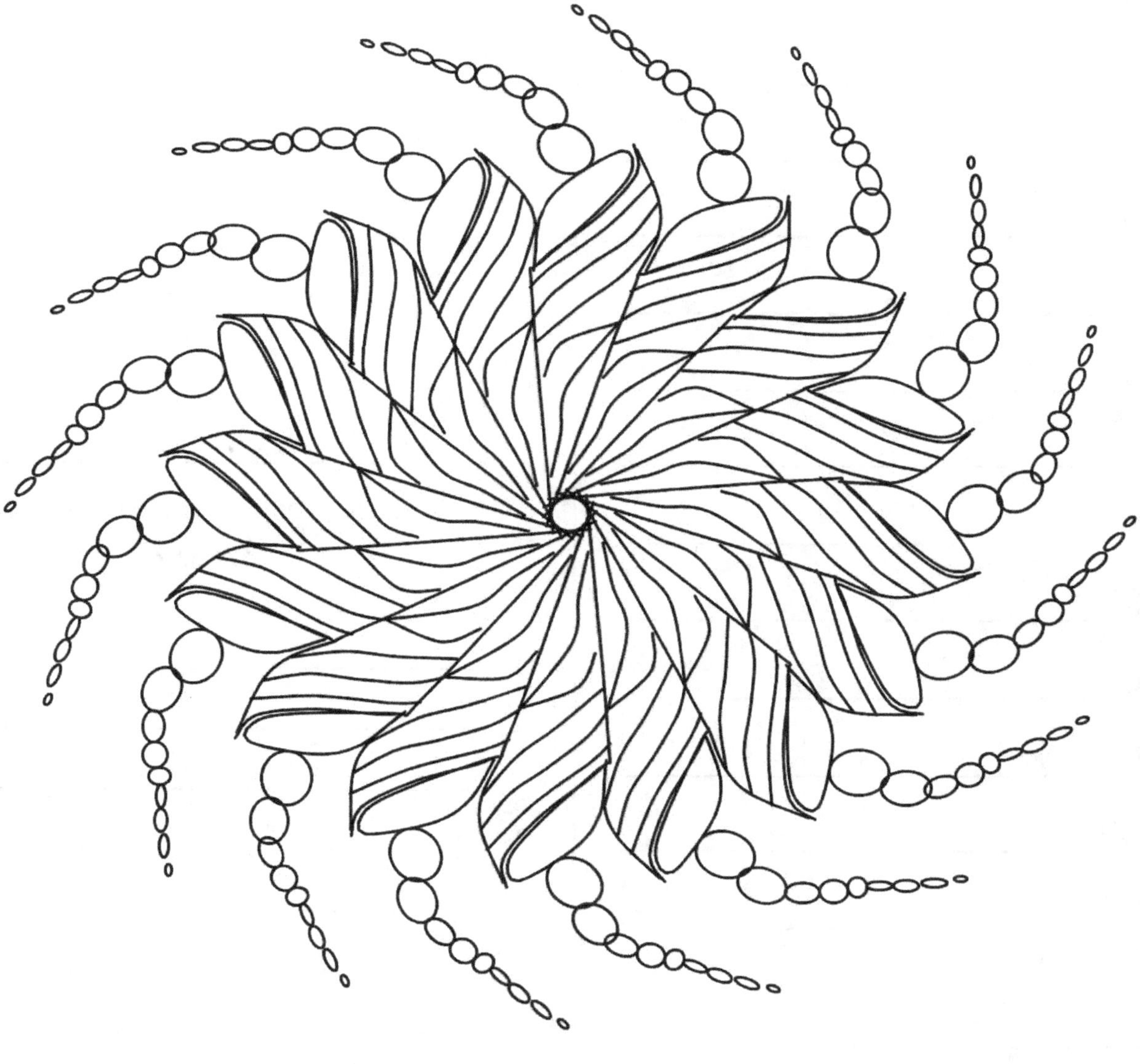

Day Thirty-two ______

5:00 ____________________
6:00 ____________________
7:00 ____________________
8:00 ____________________
9:00 ____________________
10:00 ____________________
11:00 ____________________
Noon ____________________
1:00 ____________________
2:00 ____________________
3:00 ____________________
4:00 ____________________
5:00 ____________________
6:00 ____________________
7:00 ____________________
8:00 ____________________
9:00 ____________________
10:00 ____________________
11:00 ____________________
Midnight ____________________

top priorities for today

____
____
____
____

Today's victories

What does it mean to be fervent?

____
____
____
____
____
____
____

The Stella Society Workout

Exercise	Set 1	Set 2	Set 3	Set 4	Set 5	notes

Time started: ____________ Time ended: _____________

Location: ____

Feelings before training: ☺ 😑 ☹ 😝 😠 😕 😇 😎

Feelings after training ☺ 😑 ☹ 😝 😠 😕 😇 😎

NUTRITION

Meal 1

time eaten: _________

Meal 2

time eaten: _________

Meal 3

time eaten: _________

Meal 4

time eaten: _________

Meal 5

time eaten: _________

Hydration

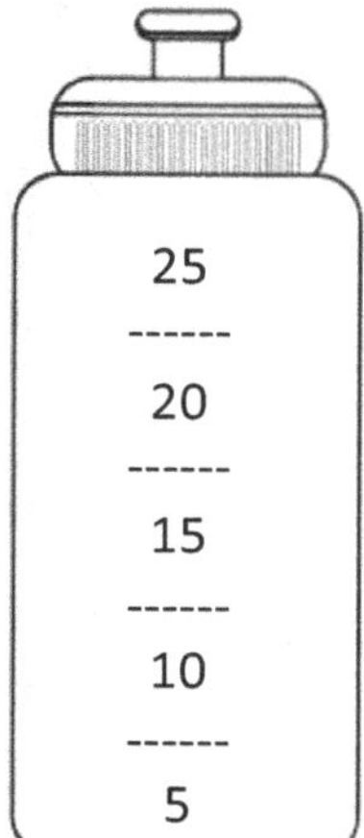

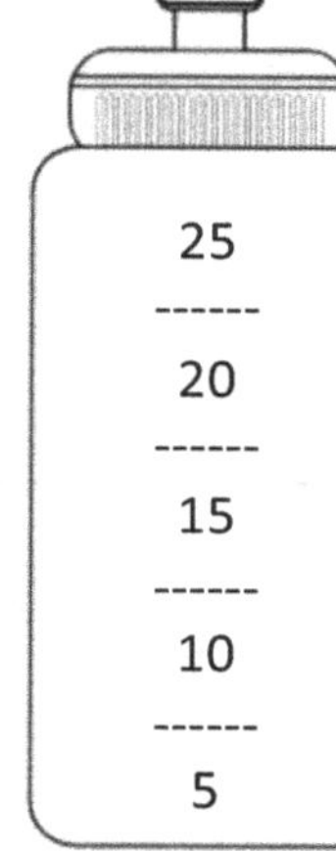

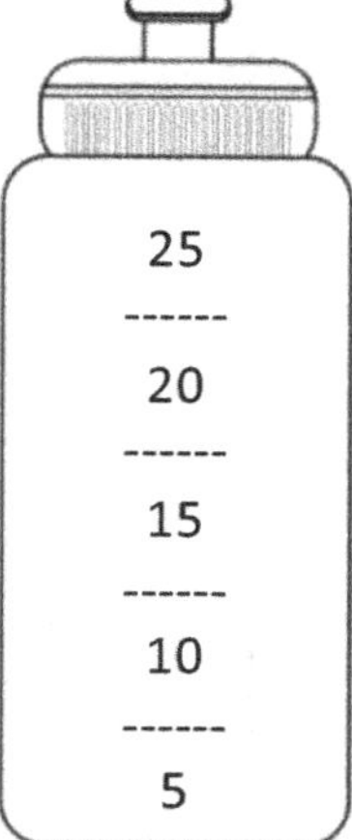

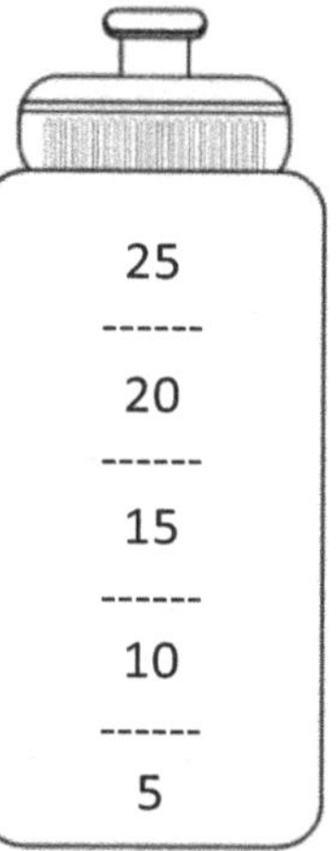

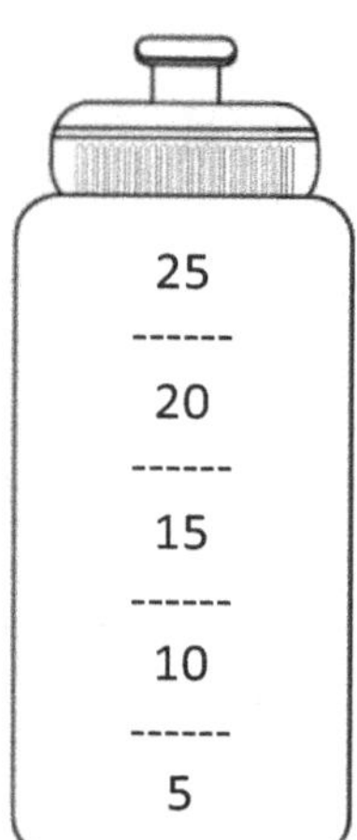

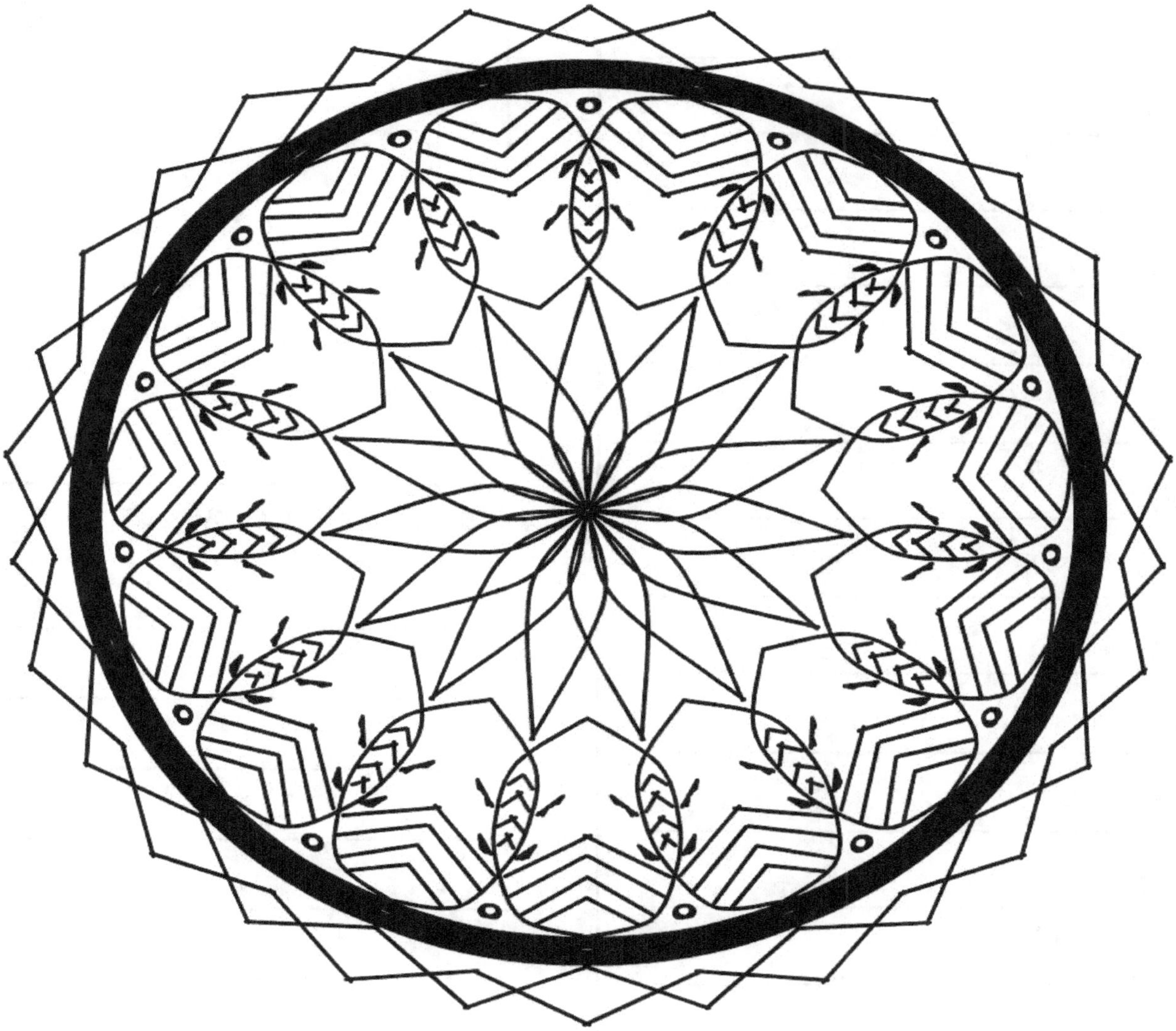

Day Thirty-three ______

5:00 ______
6:00 ______
7:00 ______
8:00 ______
9:00 ______
10:00 ______
11:00 ______
Noon ______
1:00 ______
2:00 ______
3:00 ______
4:00 ______
5:00 ______
6:00 ______
7:00 ______
8:00 ______
9:00 ______
10:00 ______
11:00 ______
Midnight ______

top priorities for today

______
______
______
______
______

Today's victories

How are you glowing today?

______
______
______
______
______
______
______
______

The Stella Society Workout

Exercise	Set 1	Set 2	Set 3	Set 4	Set 5	notes

Time started: ____________ Time ended: _____________

Location: ____

Feelings before training:

Feelings after training

NUTRITION

Meal 1

time eaten: _________

Meal 2

time eaten: _________

Meal 3

time eaten: _________

Meal 4

time eaten: _________

Meal 5

time eaten: _________

Hydration

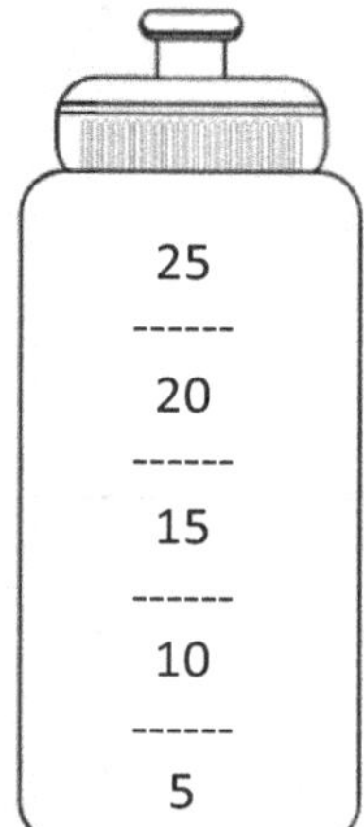

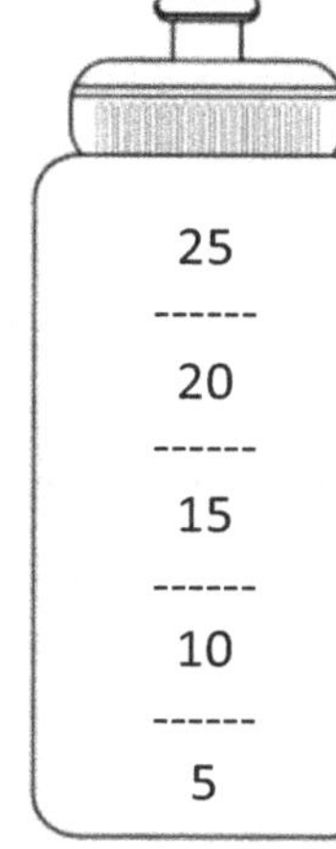

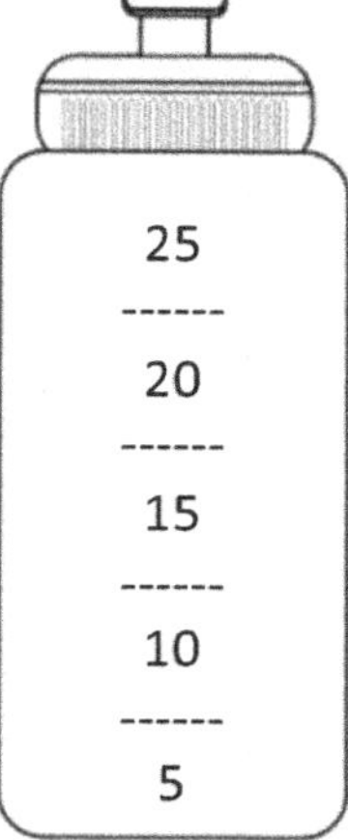

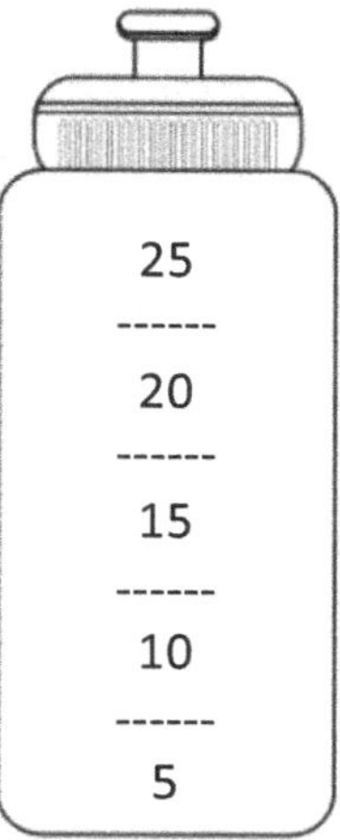

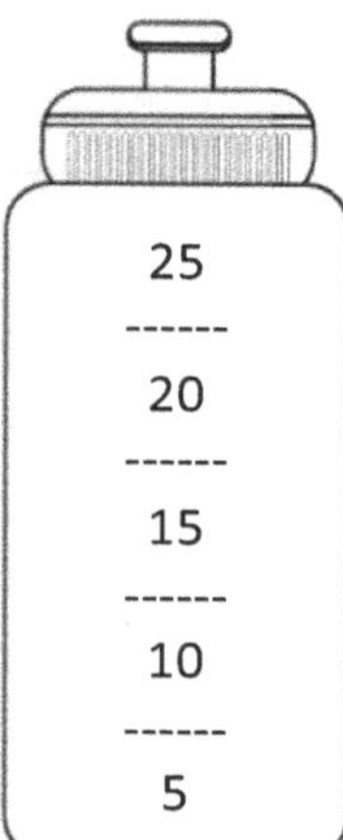

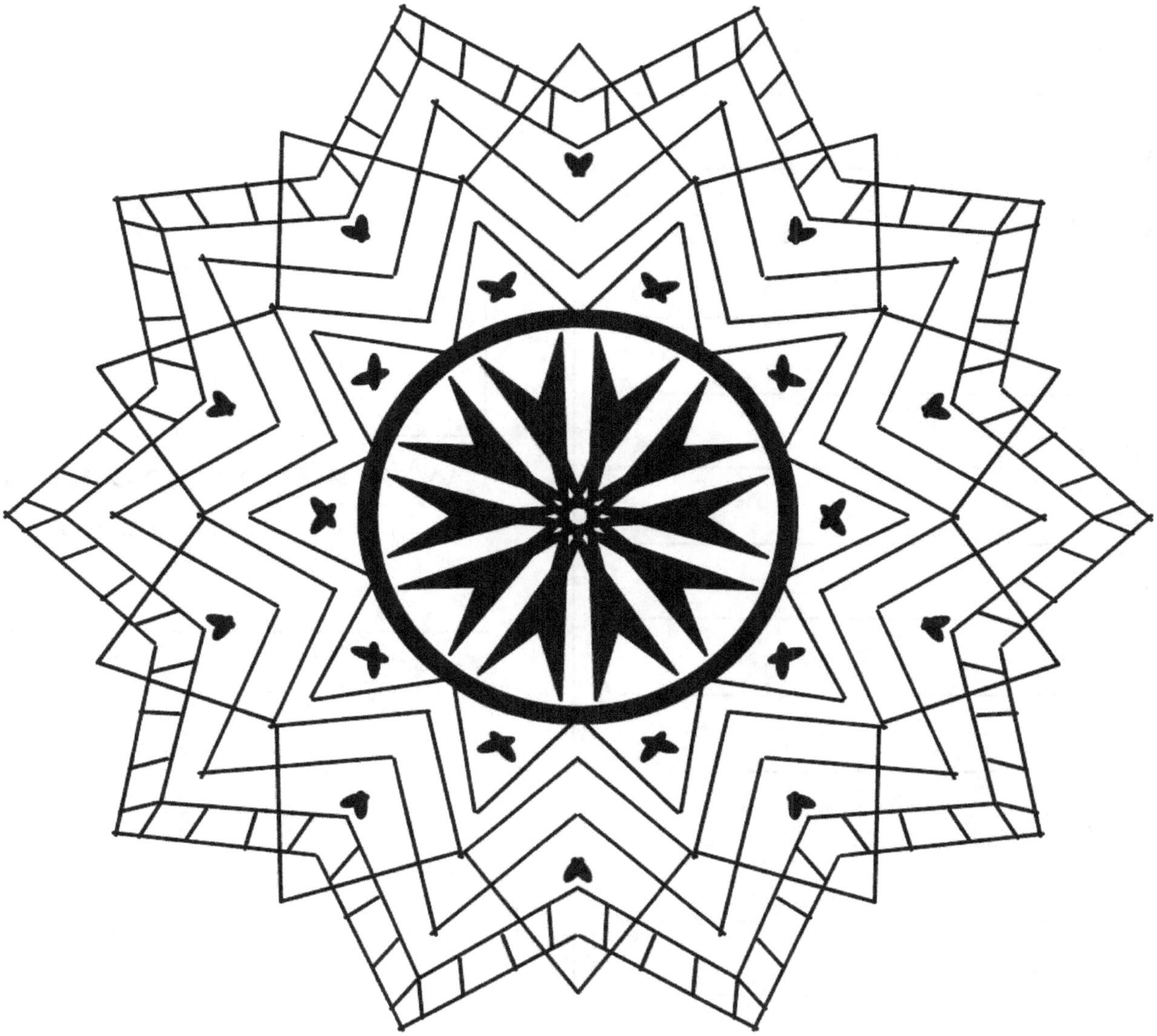

Day Thirty-four ______

5:00 ____________________

6:00 ____________________

7:00 ____________________

8:00 ____________________

9:00 ____________________

10:00 ____________________

11:00 ____________________

Noon ____________________

1:00 ____________________

2:00 ____________________

3:00 ____________________

4:00 ____________________

5:00 ____________________

6:00 ____________________

7:00 ____________________

8:00 ____________________

9:00 ____________________

10:00 ____________________

11:00 ____________________

Midnight ____________________

top priorities for today

____

____

____

____

____

Today's victories

What are you dedicated to do at this moment?

____

____

____

____

____

____

____

____

The Stella Society Workout

Exercise	Set 1	Set 2	Set 3	Set 4	Set 5	notes

Time started: ____________ Time ended: _____________

Location: ____

Feelings before training: ☺ 😑 ☹ 😝 😠 😕 😇 😎

Feelings after training ☺ 😑 ☹ 😝 😠 😕 😇 😎

NUTRITION

Meal 1

time eaten: _________

Meal 2

time eaten: _________

Meal 3

time eaten: _________

Meal 4

time eaten: _________

Meal 5

time eaten: _________

Hydration

25
20
15
10
5
25
20
15
10
5
25
20
15
10
5
25
20
15
10
5
25
20
15
10
5

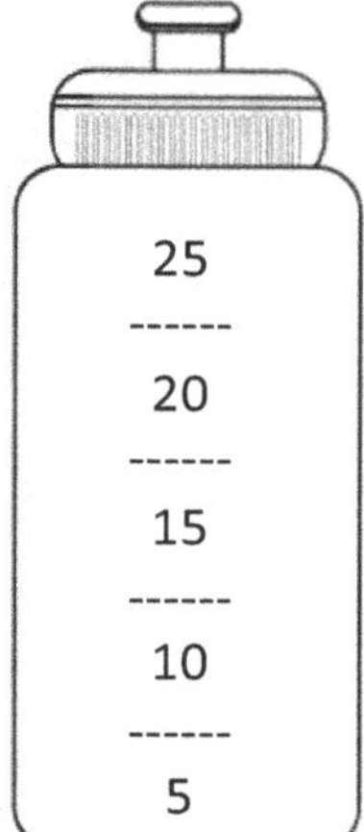

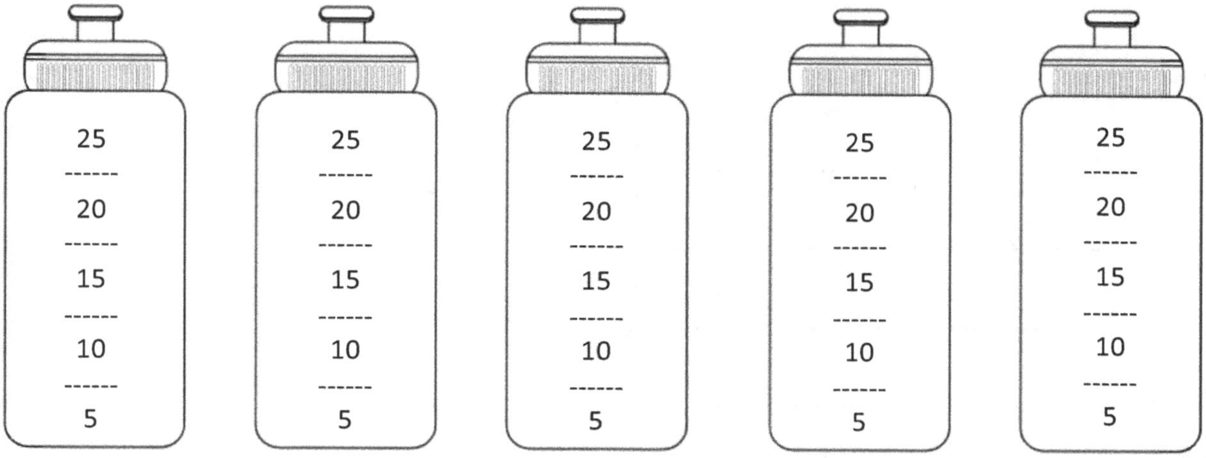

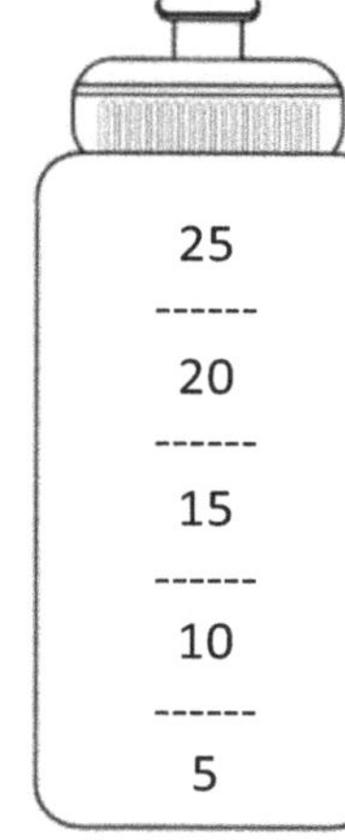

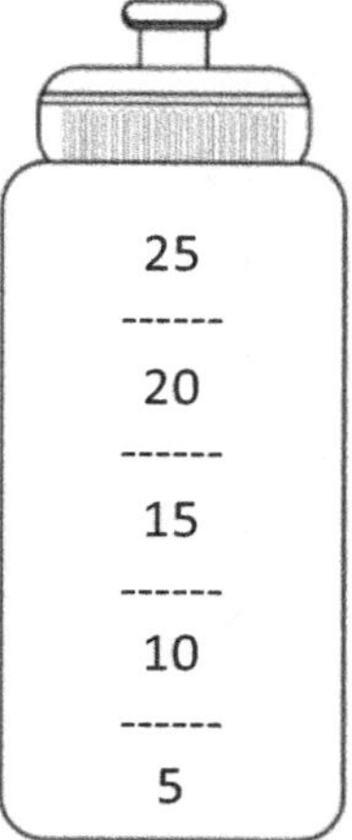

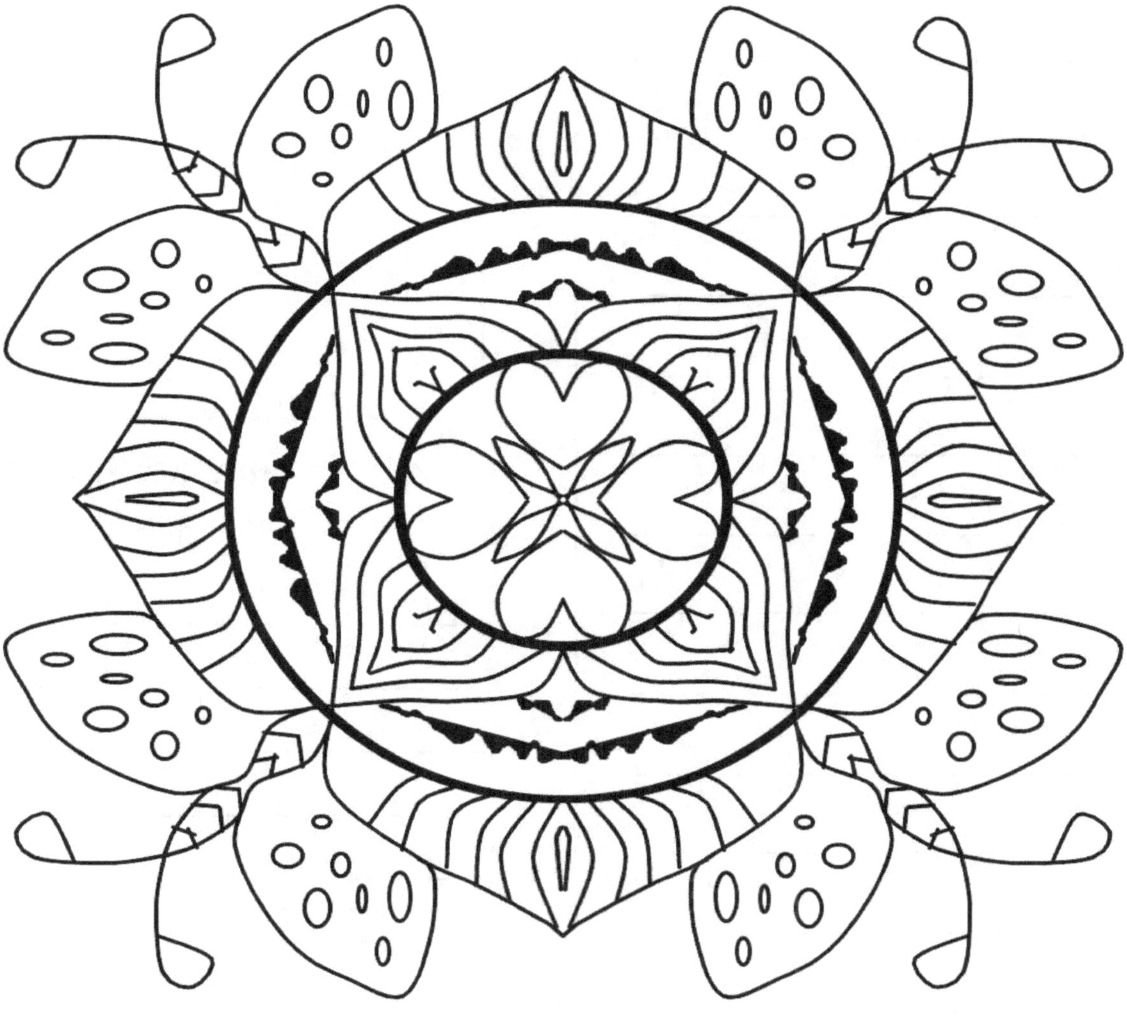

Day Thirty-five ______

5:00 ______

6:00 ______

7:00 ______

8:00 ______

9:00 ______

10:00 ______

11:00 ______

Noon ______

1:00 ______

2:00 ______

3:00 ______

4:00 ______

5:00 ______

6:00 ______

7:00 ______

8:00 ______

9:00 ______

10:00 ______

11:00 ______

Midnight ______

top priorities for today

______

______

______

______

______

Today's victories

Who is more determined than you?

______

______

______

______

______

______

______

______

The Stella Society Workout

Exercise	Set 1	Set 2	Set 3	Set 4	Set 5	notes

Time started: ____________ Time ended: _____________

Location: ____

Feelings before training:

Feelings after training

NUTRITION

Meal 1

time eaten: _________

Meal 2

time eaten: _________

Meal 3

time eaten: _________

Meal 4

time eaten: _________

Meal 5

time eaten: _________

Hydration

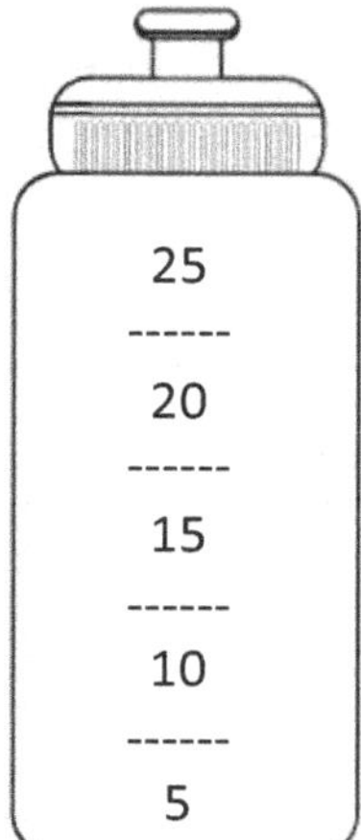

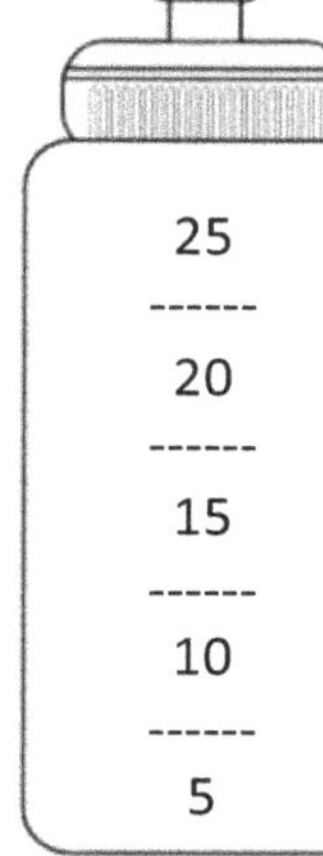

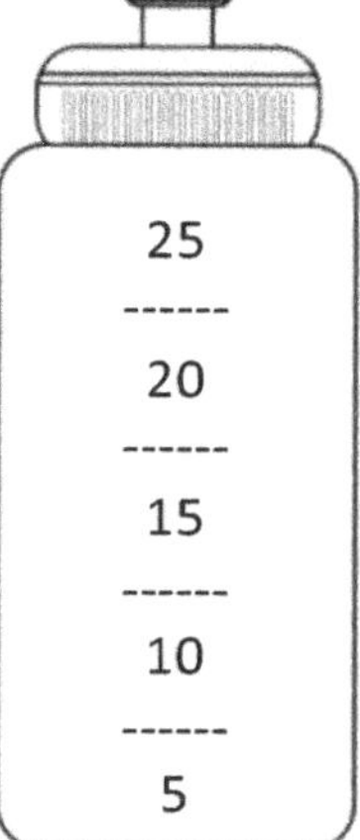

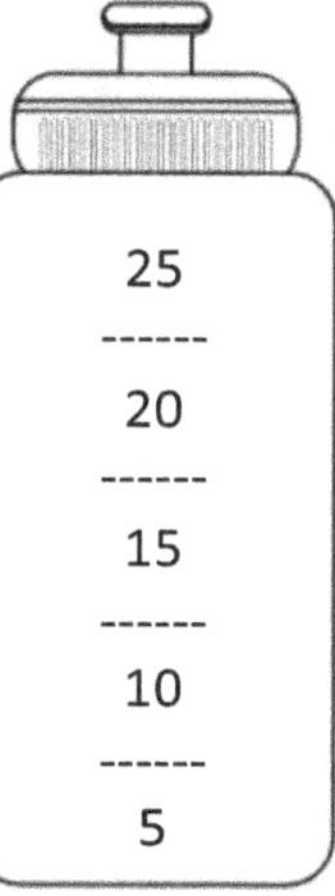

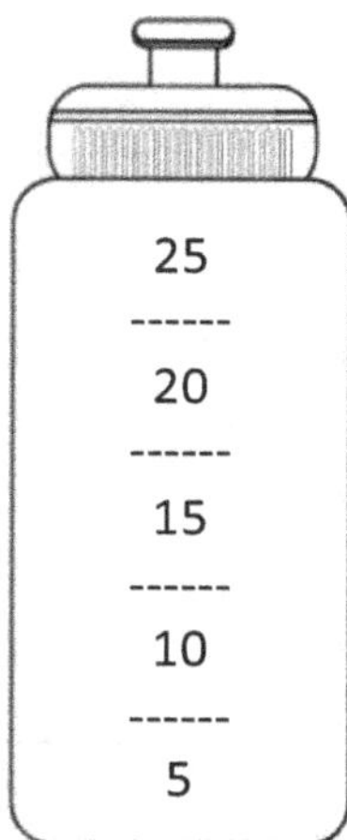

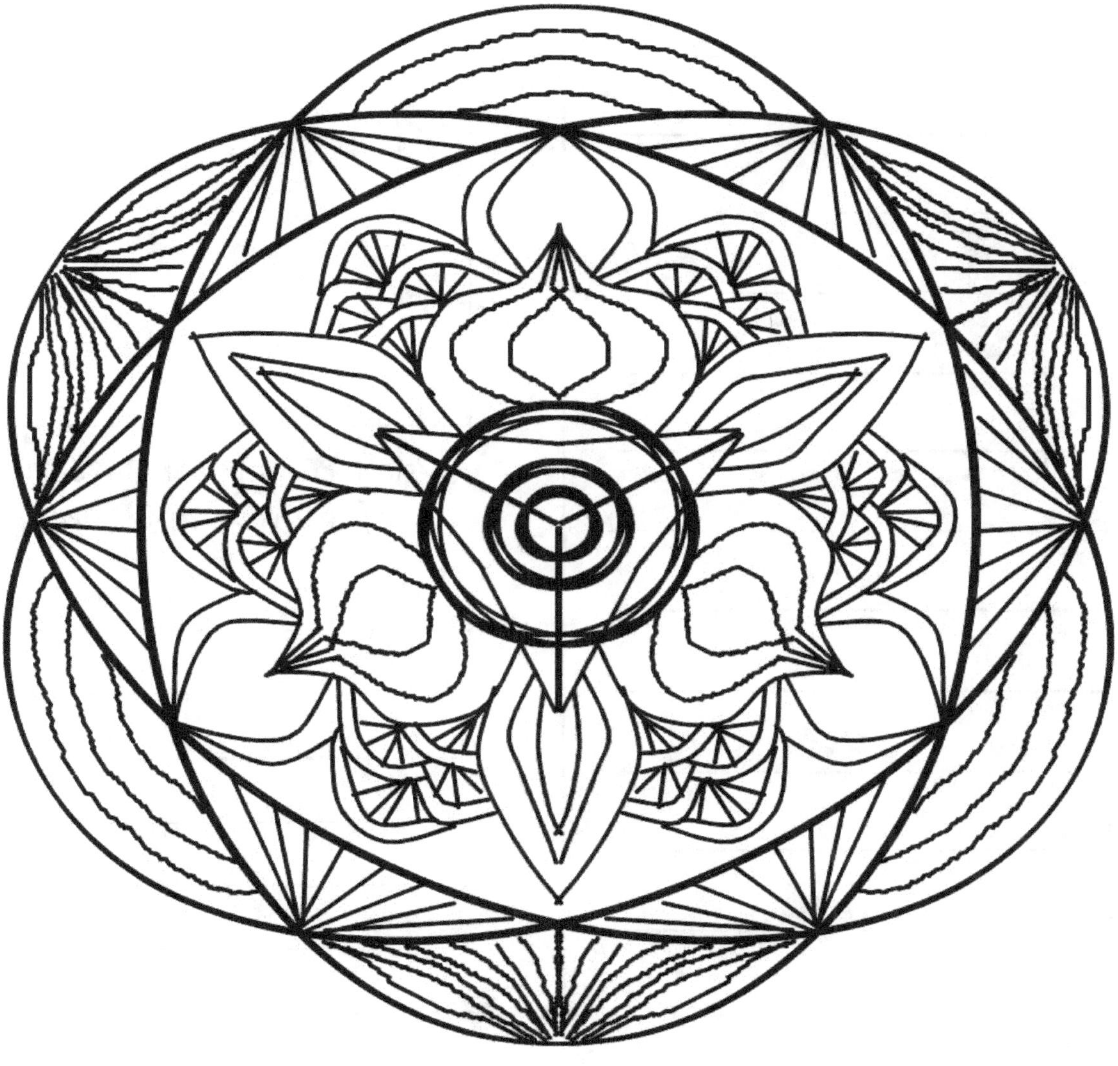

Day Thirty-six ______

5:00 ______

6:00 ______

7:00 ______

8:00 ______

9:00 ______

10:00 ______

11:00 ______

Noon ______

1:00 ______

2:00 ______

3:00 ______

4:00 ______

5:00 ______

6:00 ______

7:00 ______

8:00 ______

9:00 ______

10:00 ______

11:00 ______

Midnight ______

top priorities for today

______

______

______

______

______

Today's victories

Who needs your acceptance of change and why?

______

______

______

______

______

______

______

______

The Stella Society Workout

Exercise	Set 1	Set 2	Set 3	Set 4	Set 5	notes

Time started: ____________ Time ended: _____________

Location: ____

Feelings before training:

Feelings after training

NUTRITION

Meal 1

time eaten: _________

Meal 2

time eaten: _________

Meal 3

time eaten: _________

Meal 4

time eaten: _________

Meal 5

time eaten: _________

Hydration

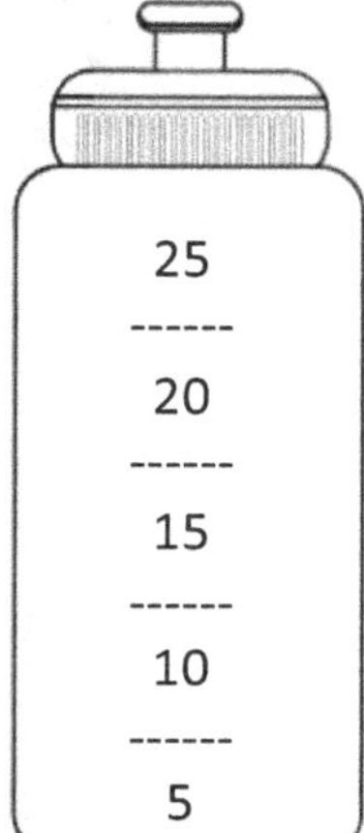

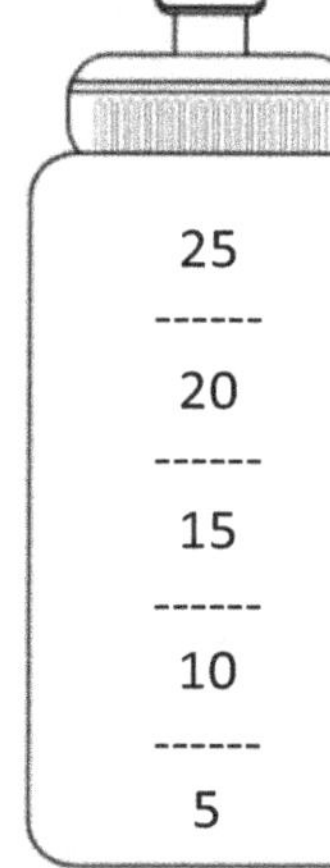

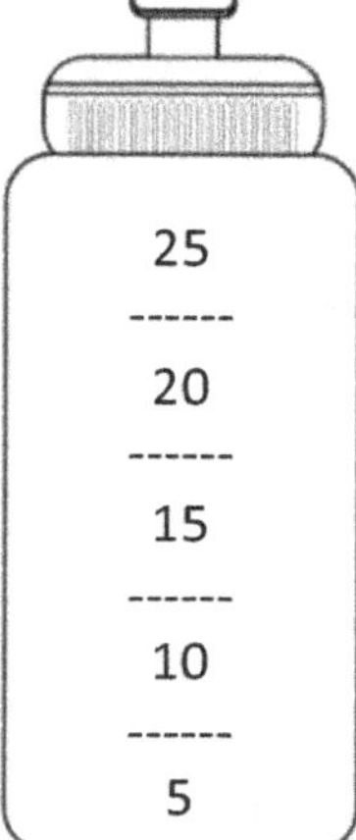

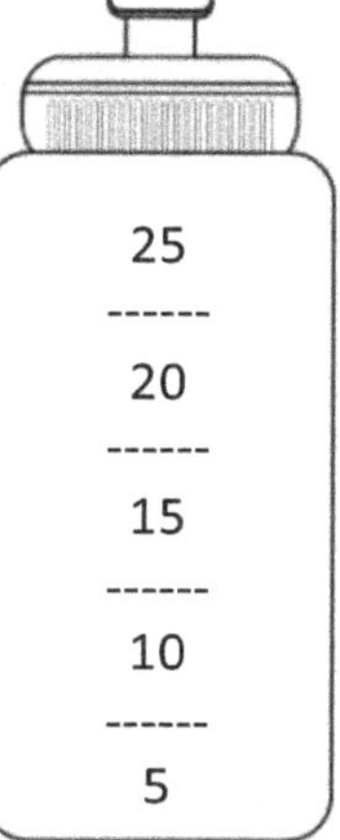

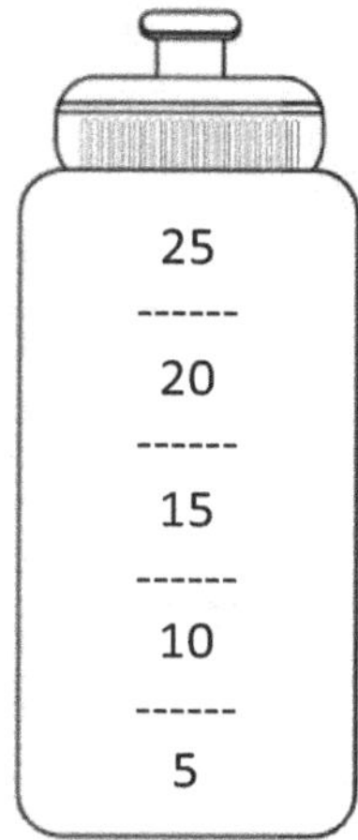

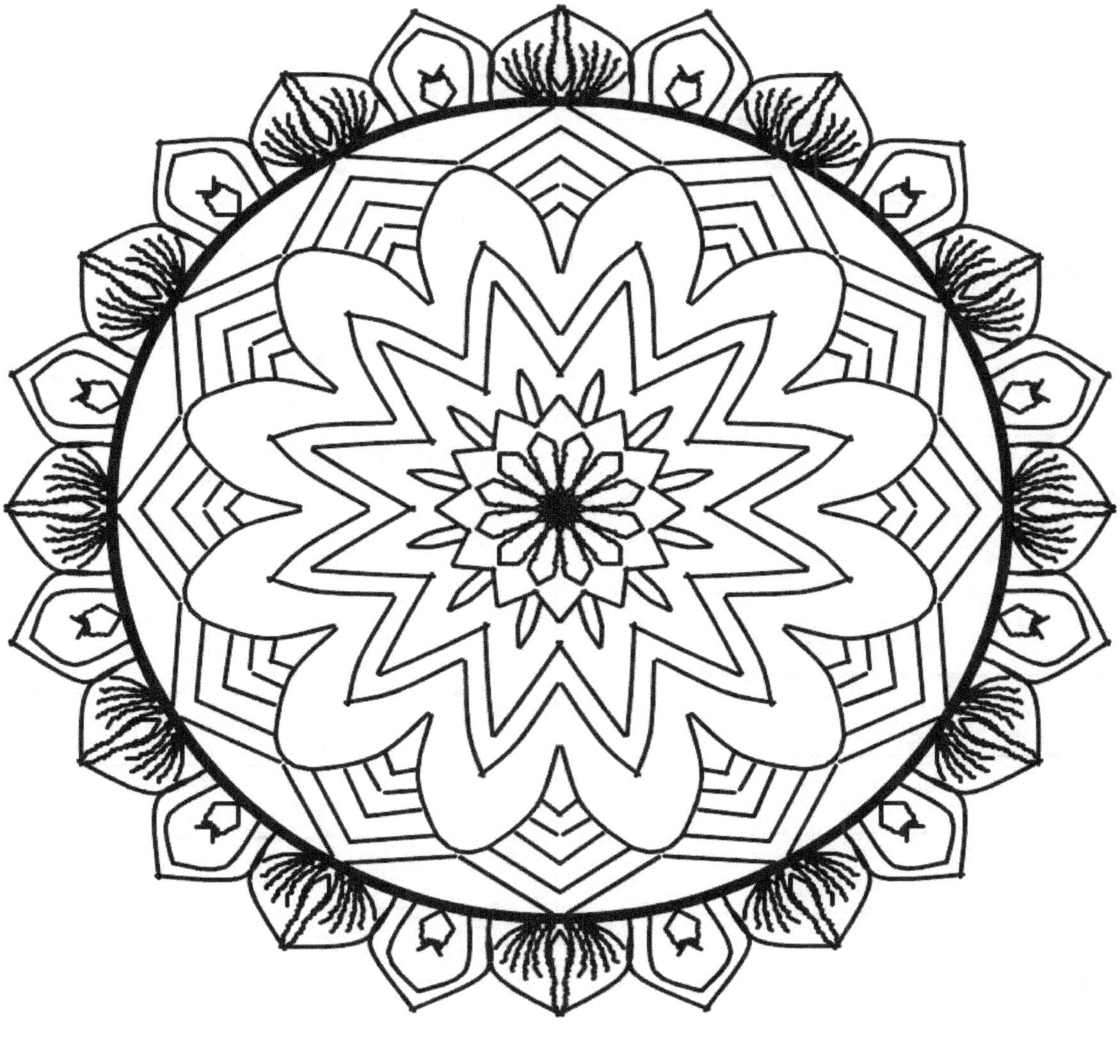

Day Thirty-seven ______

5:00 ____________________

6:00 ____________________

7:00 ____________________

8:00 ____________________

9:00 ____________________

10:00 ____________________

11:00 ____________________

Noon ____________________

1:00 ____________________

2:00 ____________________

3:00 ____________________

4:00 ____________________

5:00 ____________________

6:00 ____________________

7:00 ____________________

8:00 ____________________

9:00 ____________________

10:00 ____________________

11:00 ____________________

Midnight ____________________

top priorities for today

____

____

____

____

____

Today's victories

How will you be captivating?

____

____

____

____

____

____

____

____

The Stella Society Workout

Exercise	Set 1	Set 2	Set 3	Set 4	Set 5	notes

Time started: ____________ Time ended: _____________

Location: ____

Feelings before training:

Feelings after training

NUTRITION

Meal 1

time eaten: _________

Meal 2

time eaten: _________

Meal 3

time eaten: _________

Meal 4

time eaten: _________

Meal 5

time eaten: _________

Hydration

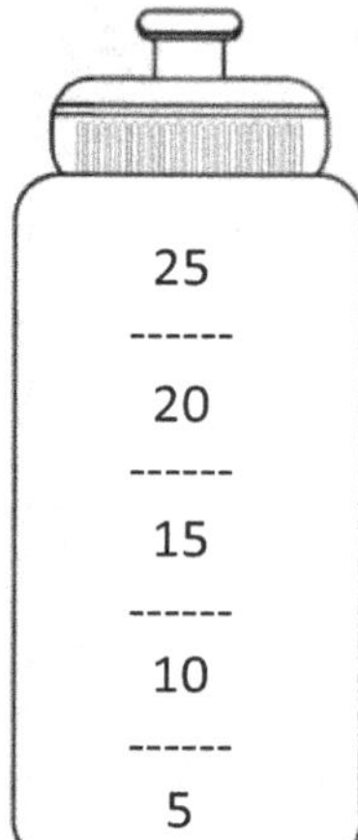

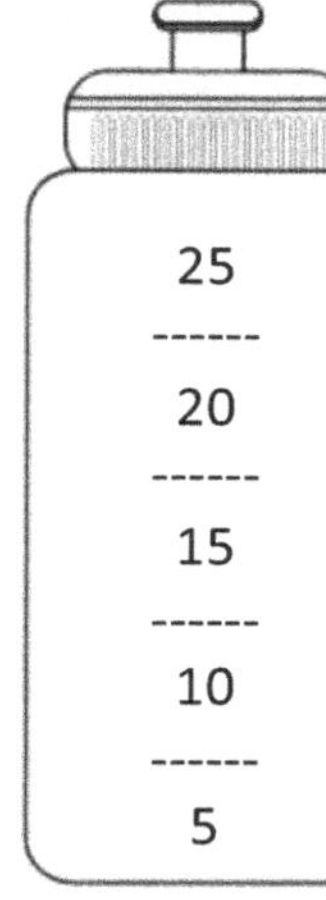

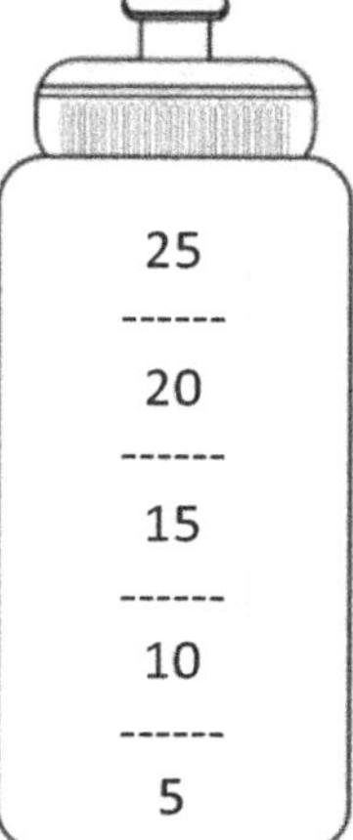

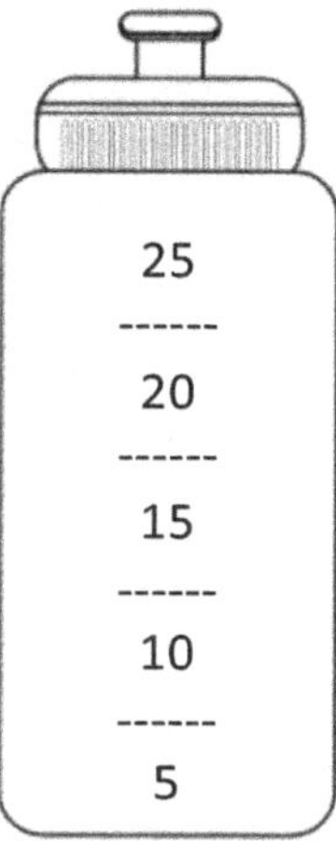

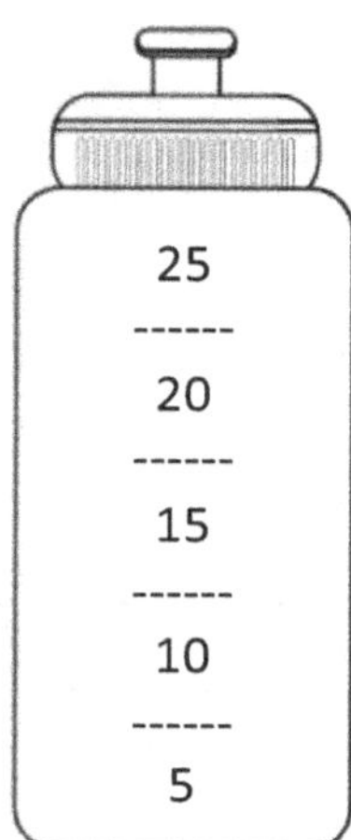

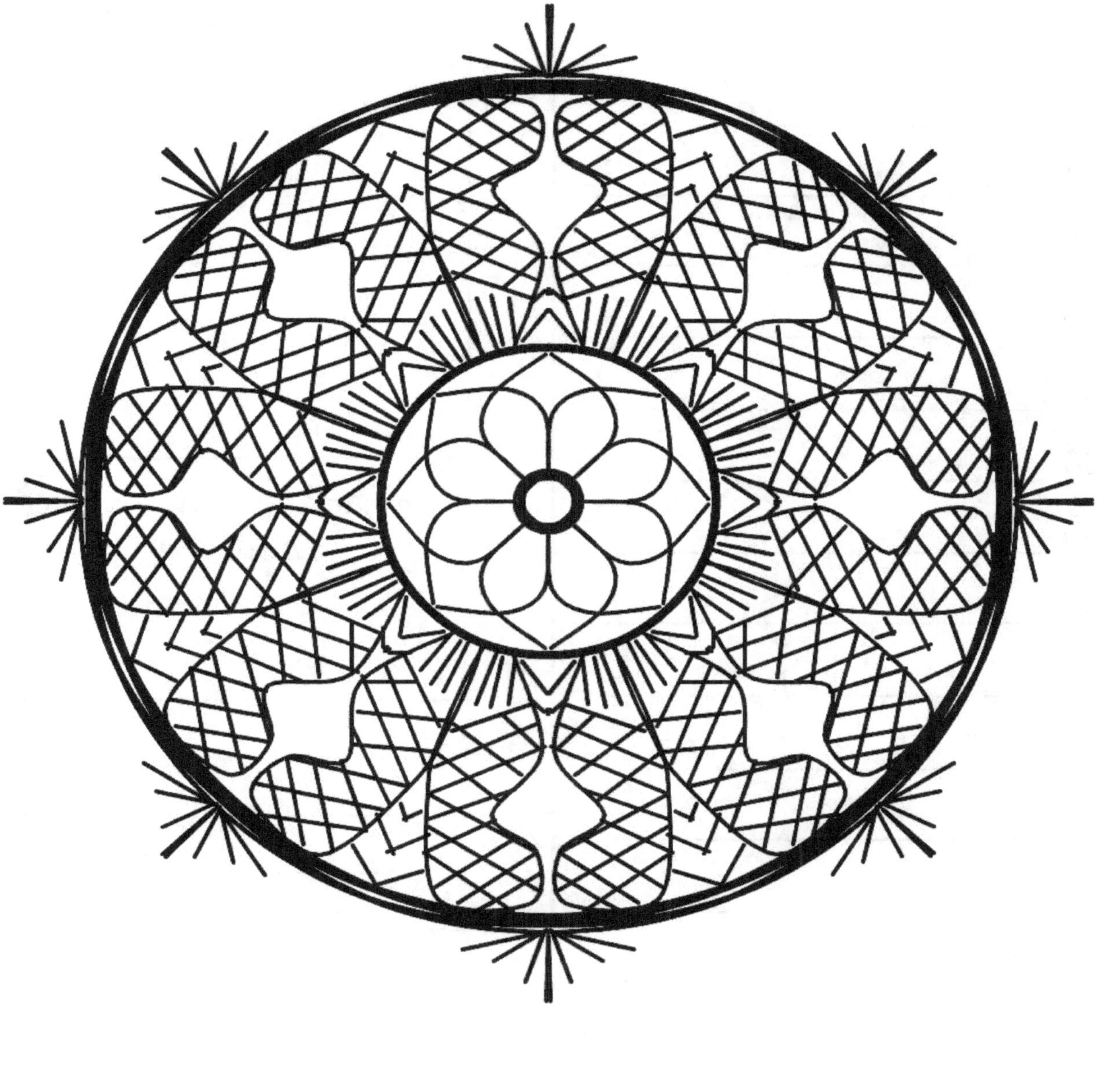

Day Thirty-eight ______

5:00 ____________________
6:00 ____________________
7:00 ____________________
8:00 ____________________
9:00 ____________________
10:00 ____________________
11:00 ____________________
Noon ____________________
1:00 ____________________
2:00 ____________________
3:00 ____________________
4:00 ____________________
5:00 ____________________
6:00 ____________________
7:00 ____________________
8:00 ____________________
9:00 ____________________
10:00 ____________________
11:00 ____________________
Midnight ____________________

top priorities for today

____
____
____
____
____

Today's victories

What does it mean to be alluring?

____
____
____
____
____
____
____
____

The Stella Society Workout

Exercise	Set 1	Set 2	Set 3	Set 4	Set 5	notes

Time started: ____________ Time ended: _____________

Location: ____

Feelings before training: ☺ 😑 ☹ 😝 😠 😕 😇 😎

Feelings after training ☺ 😑 ☹ 😝 😠 😕 😇 😎

NUTRITION

Meal 1

time eaten: _________

Meal 2

time eaten: _________

Meal 3

time eaten: _________

Meal 4

time eaten: _________

Meal 5

time eaten: _________

Hydration

25

20

15

10

5
25

20

15

10

5
25

20

15

10

5
25

20

15

10

5
25

20

15

10

5

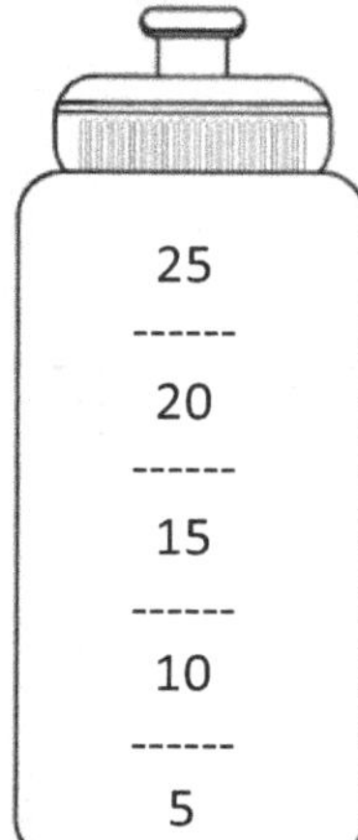

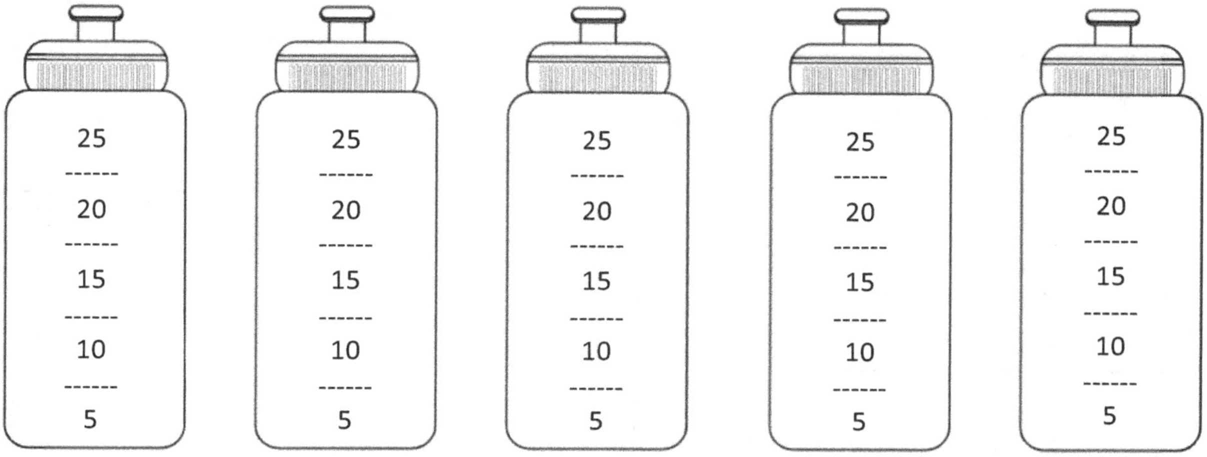

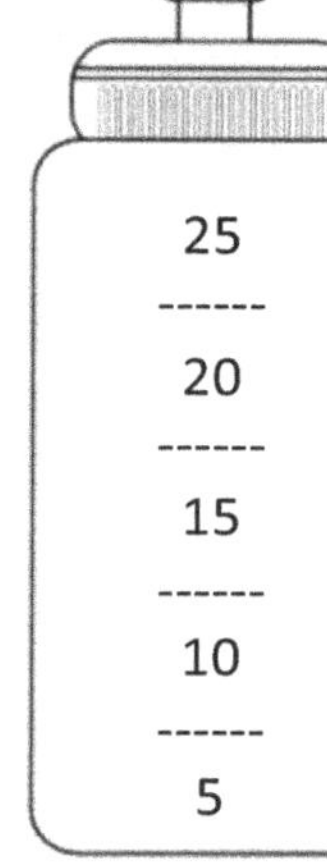

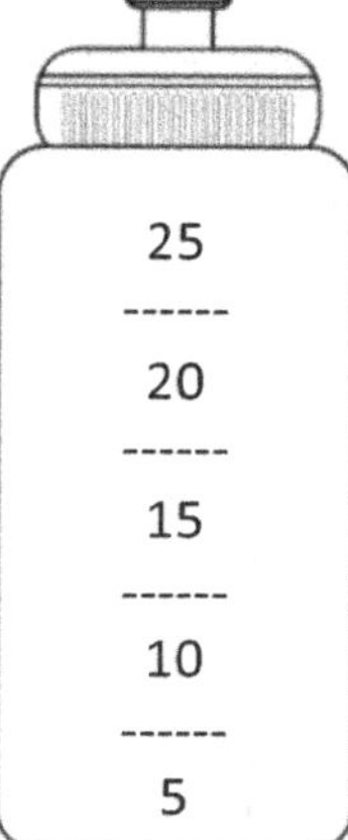

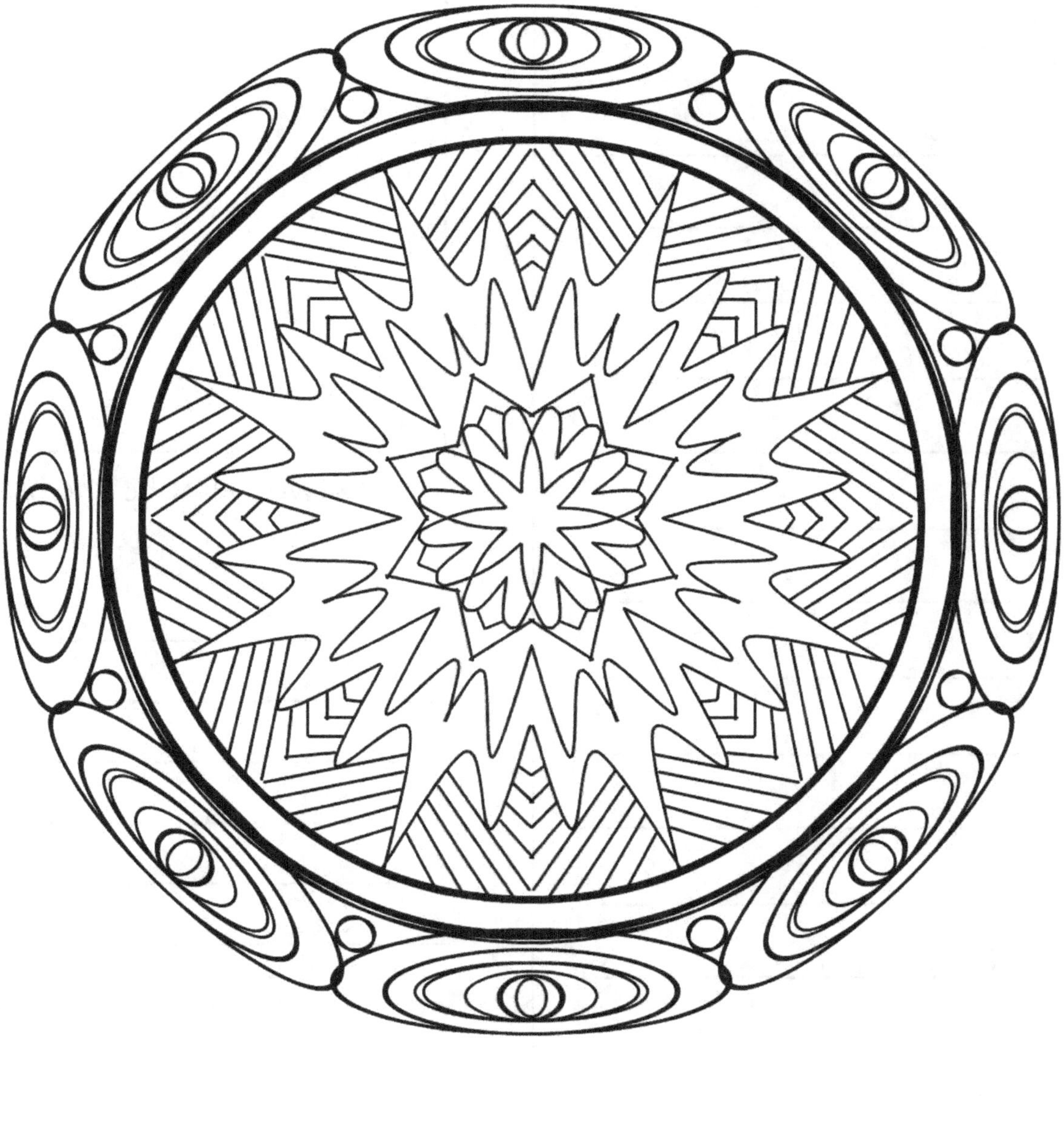

Day Thirty-nine ______

5:00 ______
6:00 ______
7:00 ______
8:00 ______
9:00 ______
10:00 ______
11:00 ______
Noon ______
1:00 ______
2:00 ______
3:00 ______
4:00 ______
5:00 ______
6:00 ______
7:00 ______
8:00 ______
9:00 ______
10:00 ______
11:00 ______
Midnight ______

top priorities for today

______
______
______
______
______

Today's victories

How will you be the best version of you?

______
______
______
______
______
______
______
______

The Stella Society Workout

Exercise	Set 1	Set 2	Set 3	Set 4	Set 5	notes

Time started: ____________ Time ended: _____________

Location: ____

Feelings before training:

Feelings after training

NUTRITION

Meal 1

time eaten: _________

Meal 2

time eaten: _________

Meal 3

time eaten: _________

Meal 4

time eaten: _________

Meal 5

time eaten: _________

Hydration

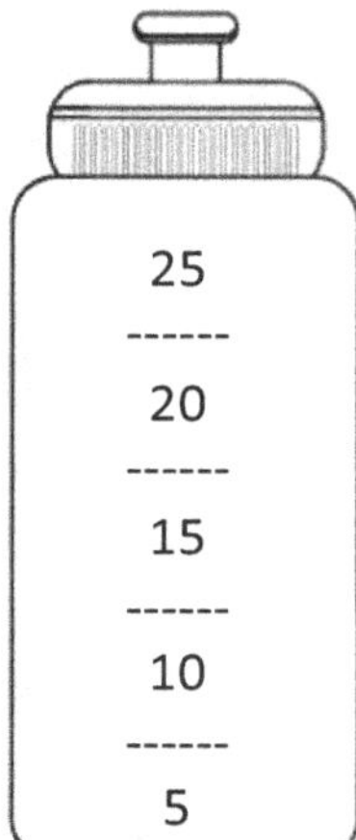

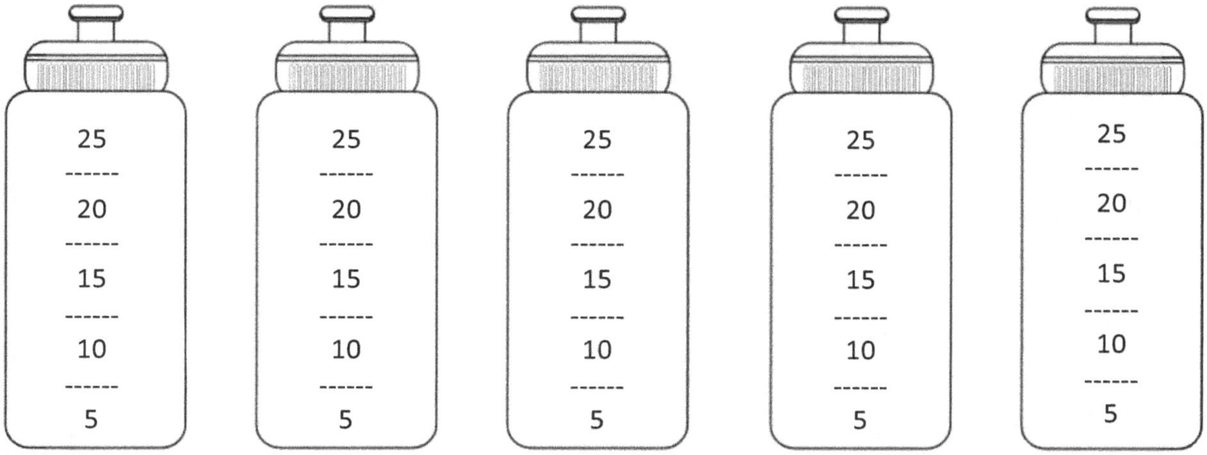

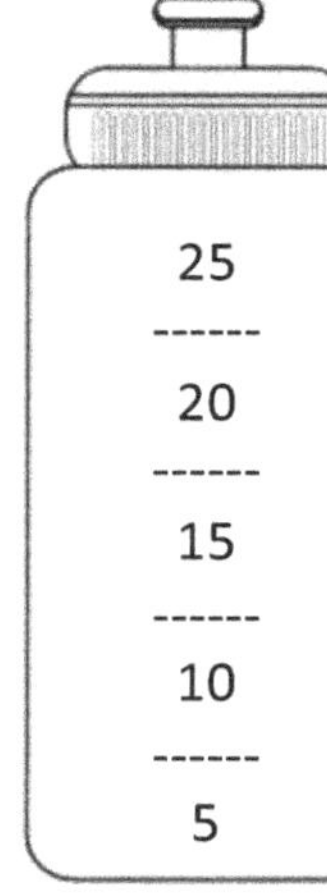

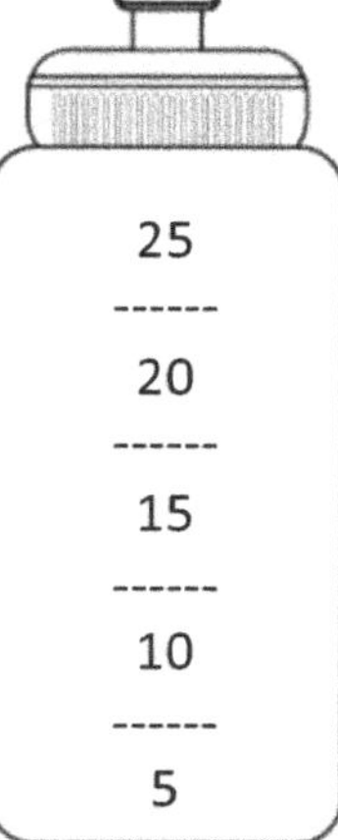

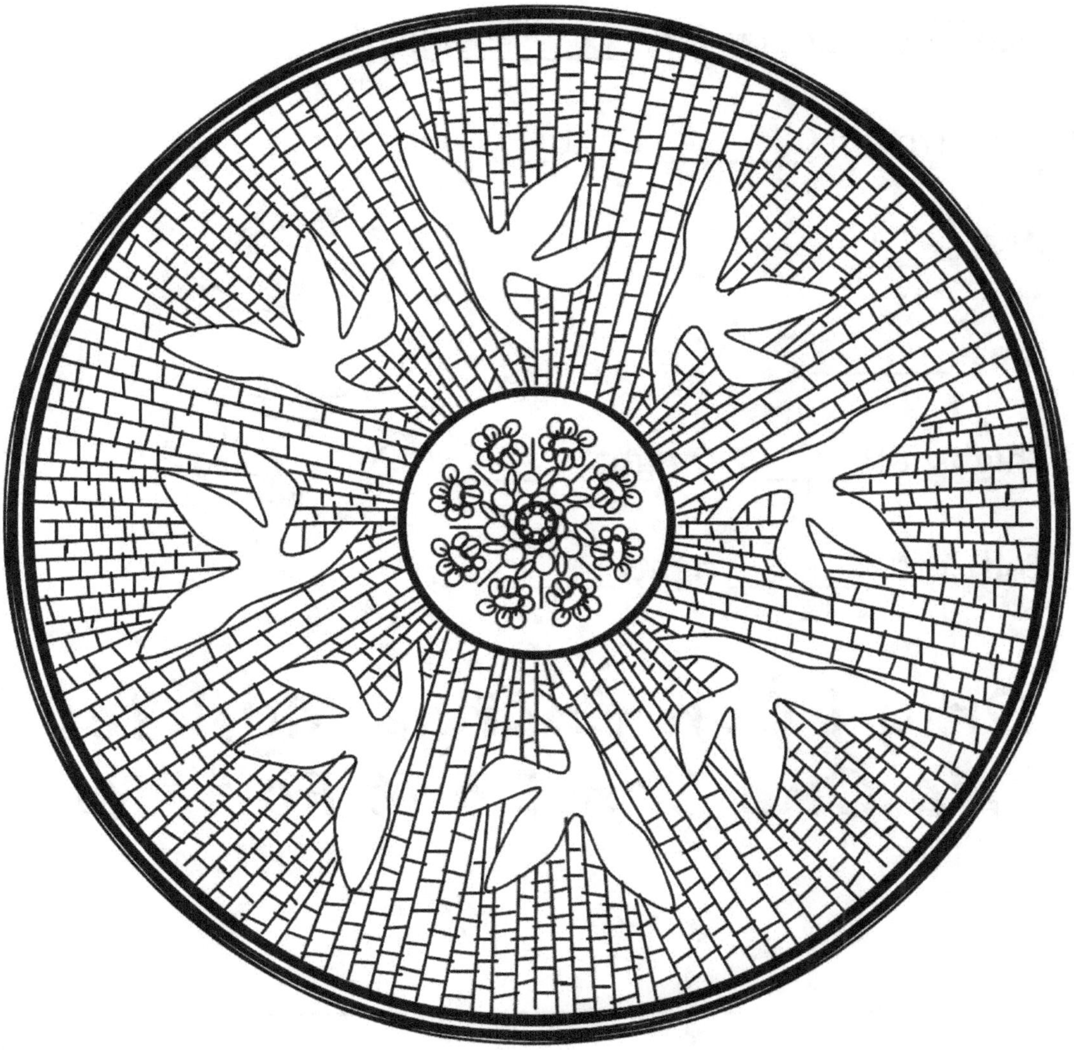

25

20

15

10

5

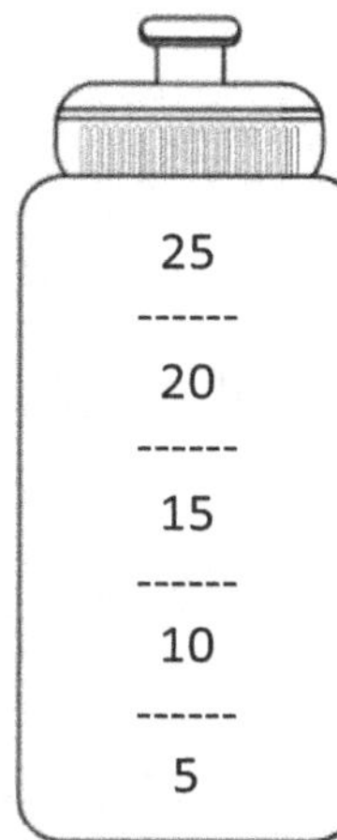

Measurements

P R O G R E S S

C H E C K

DATE: __________

Weight: ______

Neck ______

Shoulders ______

Chest ______

Bicep / upper arm left _______ right ______

Forearm left _______ right ______

Waist ______

Hips ______

Thighs left _______ right ______

Calf left _______ right ______

Only I Can Change My Life, No One Can Do It For Me!

Day Forty ______

5:00 ____________________
6:00 ____________________
7:00 ____________________
8:00 ____________________
9:00 ____________________
10:00 ____________________
11:00 ____________________
Noon ____________________
1:00 ____________________
2:00 ____________________
3:00 ____________________
4:00 ____________________
5:00 ____________________
6:00 ____________________
7:00 ____________________
8:00 ____________________
9:00 ____________________
10:00 ____________________
11:00 ____________________
Midnight ____________________

top priorities for today

____
____
____
____
____

Today's victories

Do you believe in magic or miracles?

____
____
____
____
____
____
____
____

The Stella Society Workout

Exercise	Set 1	Set 2	Set 3	Set 4	Set 5	notes

Time started: ____________ Time ended: _____________

Location: ____

Feelings before training:

Feelings after training

NUTRITION

Meal 1

time eaten: _________

Meal 2

time eaten: _________

Meal 3

time eaten: _________

Meal 4

time eaten: _________

Meal 5

time eaten: _________

Hydration

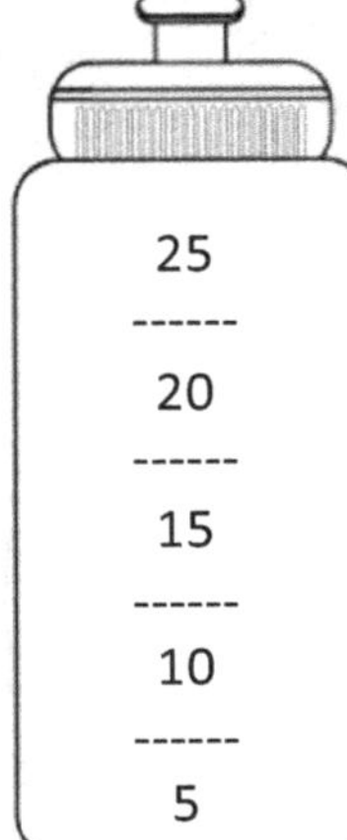

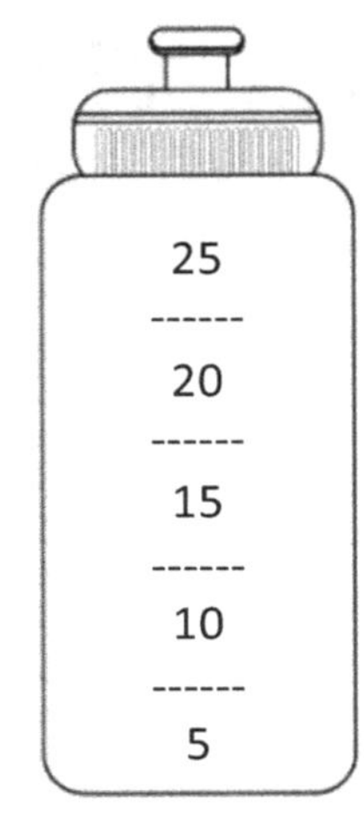

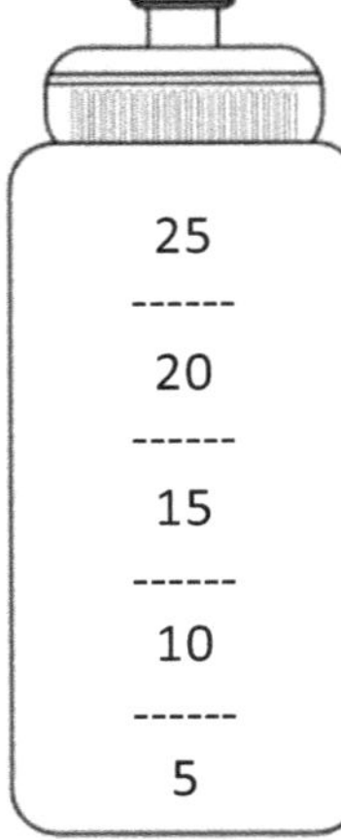

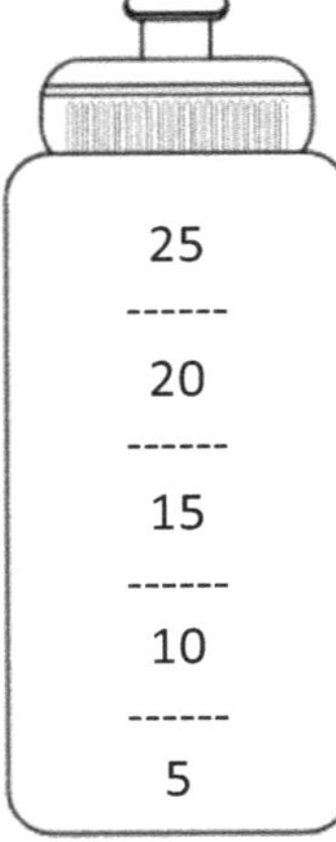

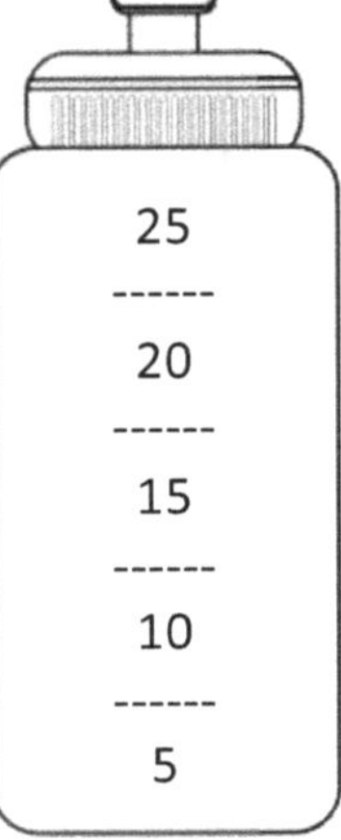

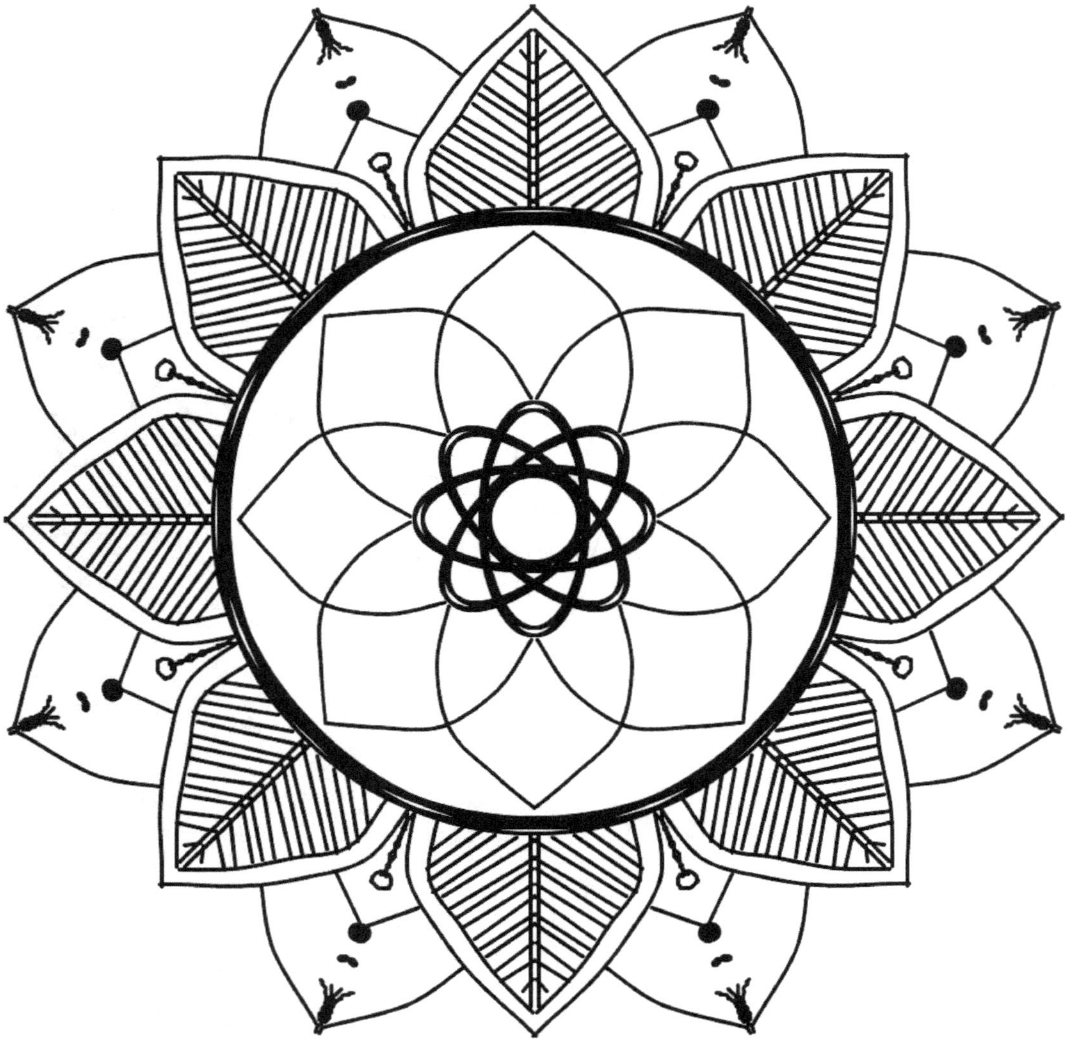

Day Forty-one ______

5:00 ____________________

6:00 ____________________

7:00 ____________________

8:00 ____________________

9:00 ____________________

10:00 ____________________

11:00 ____________________

Noon ____________________

1:00 ____________________

2:00 ____________________

3:00 ____________________

4:00 ____________________

5:00 ____________________

6:00 ____________________

7:00 ____________________

8:00 ____________________

9:00 ____________________

10:00 ____________________

11:00 ____________________

Midnight ____________________

top priorities for today

____

____

____

____

Today's victories

What is one thing you want to do forever?

____

____

____

____

____

____

____

The Stella Society Workout

Exercise	Set 1	Set 2	Set 3	Set 4	Set 5	notes

Time started: ____________ Time ended: _____________

Location: ____

Feelings before training:

Feelings after training

NUTRITION

Meal 1

time eaten: _________

Meal 2

time eaten: _________

Meal 3

time eaten: _________

Meal 4

time eaten: _________

Meal 5

time eaten: _________

Hydration

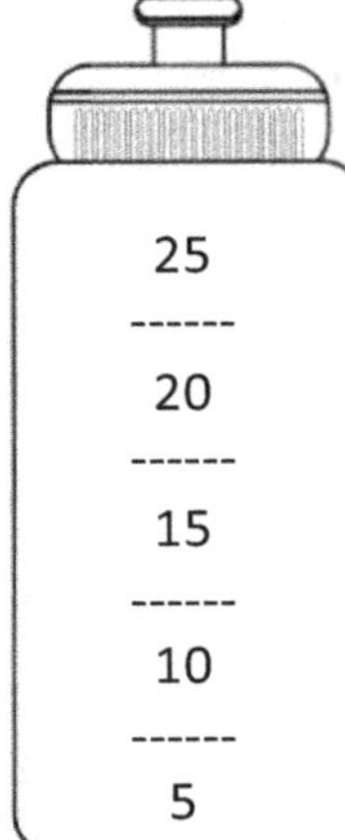

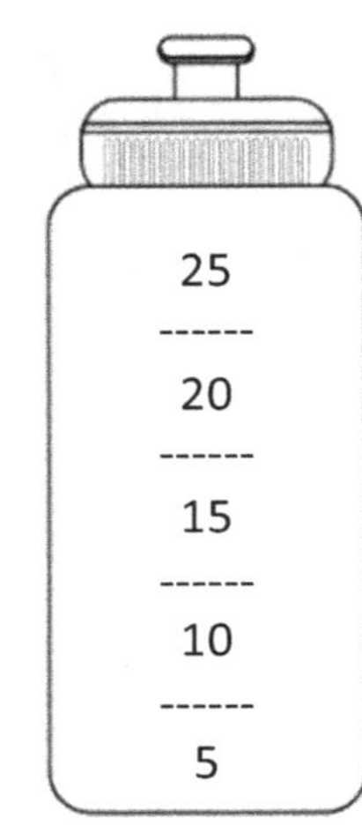

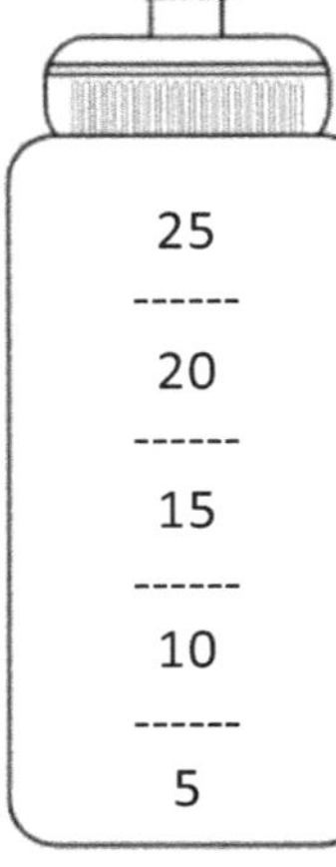

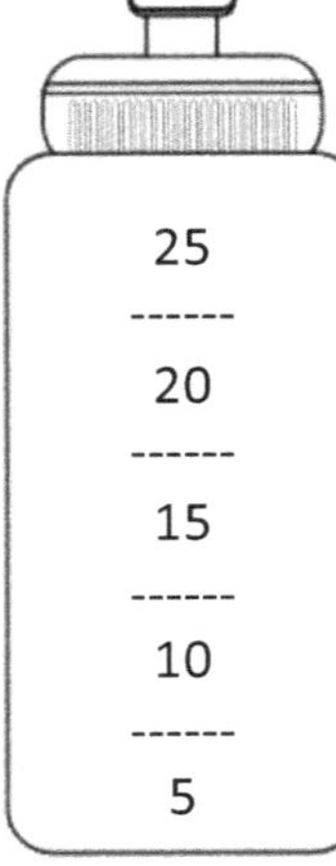

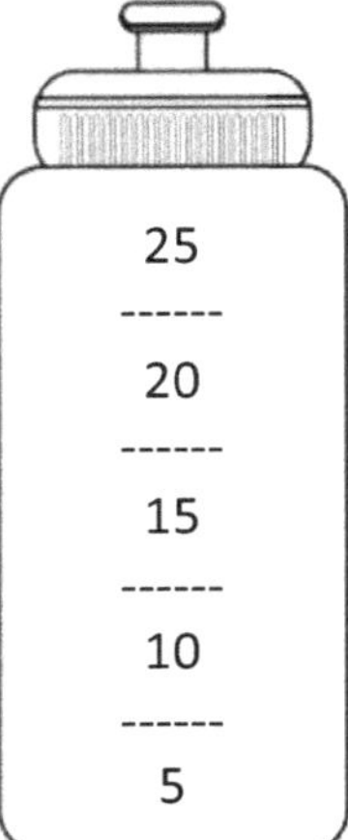

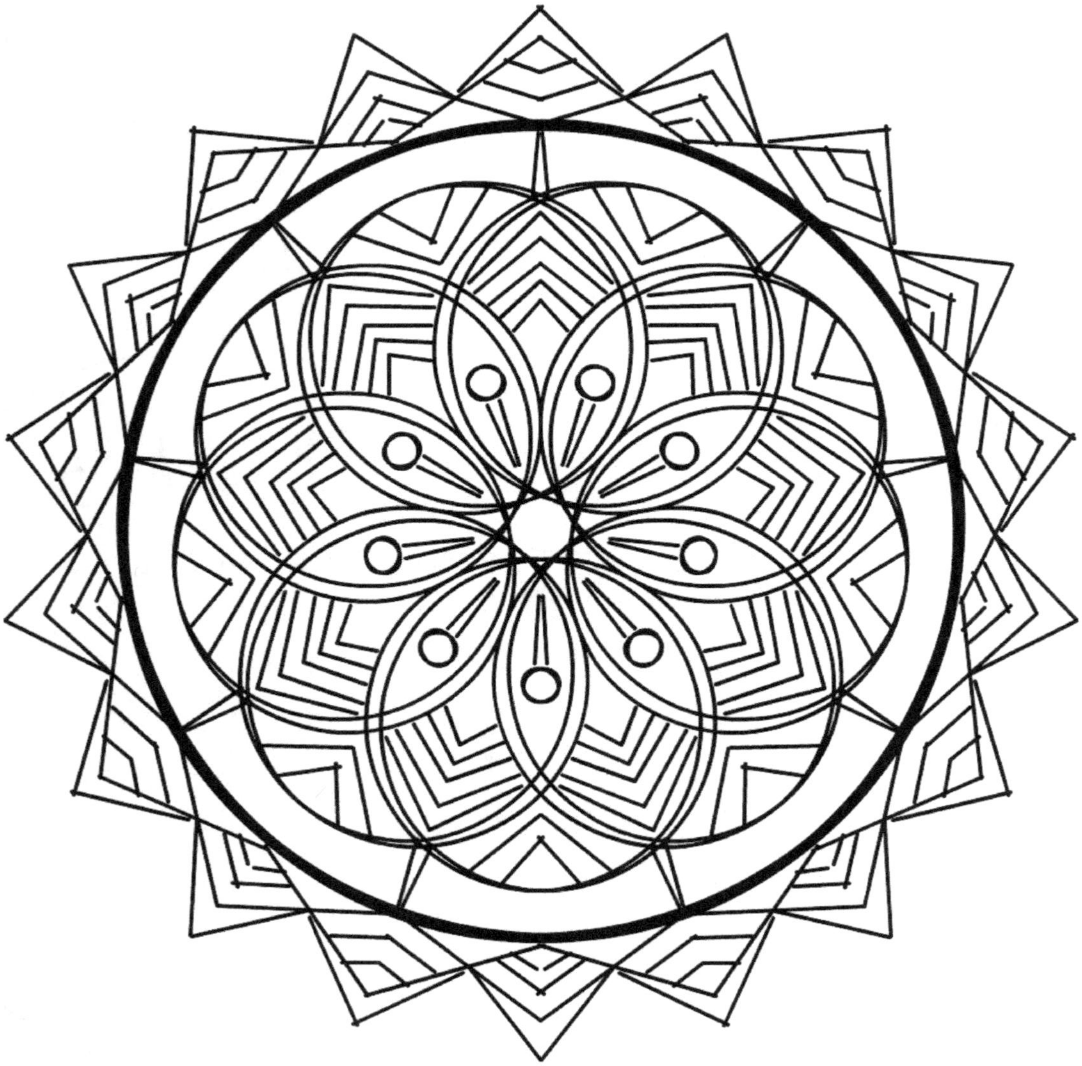

Day Forty-two ______

5:00 ______
6:00 ______
7:00 ______
8:00 ______
9:00 ______
10:00 ______
11:00 ______
Noon ______
1:00 ______
2:00 ______
3:00 ______
4:00 ______
5:00 ______
6:00 ______
7:00 ______
8:00 ______
9:00 ______
10:00 ______
11:00 ______
Midnight ______

top priorities for today

______
______
______
______
______

Today's victories

What was your biggest victory in the last 40 days?

______
______
______
______
______
______
______
______

The Stella Society Workout

Exercise	Set 1	Set 2	Set 3	Set 4	Set 5	notes

Time started: ____________ Time ended: _____________

Location: ____

Feelings before training:

Feelings after training

NUTRITION

Meal 1

time eaten: _________

Meal 2

time eaten: _________

Meal 3

time eaten: _________

Meal 4

time eaten: _________

Meal 5

time eaten: _________

Hydration

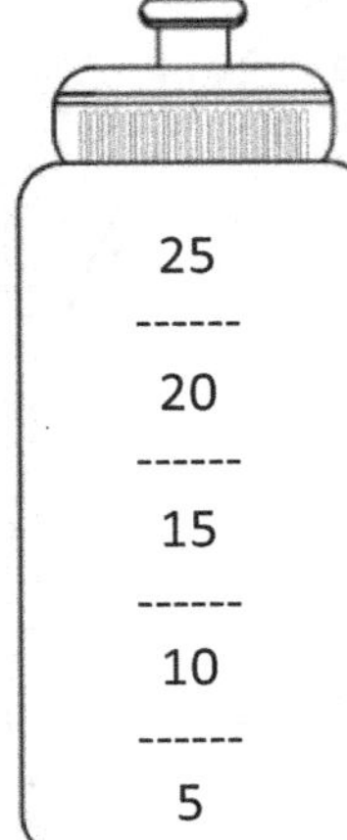

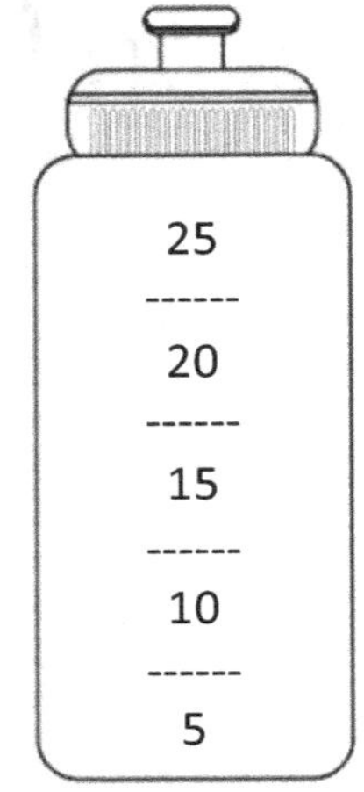

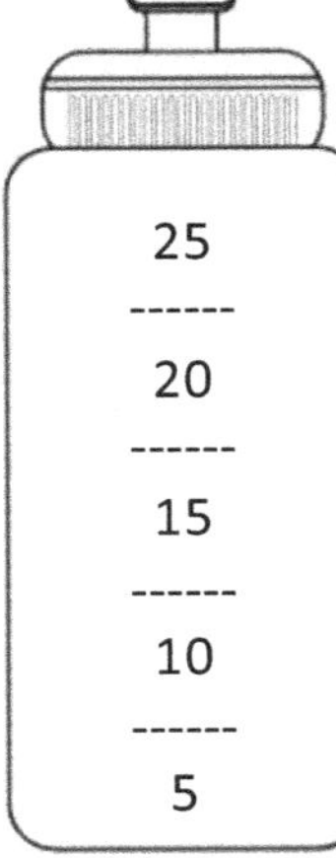

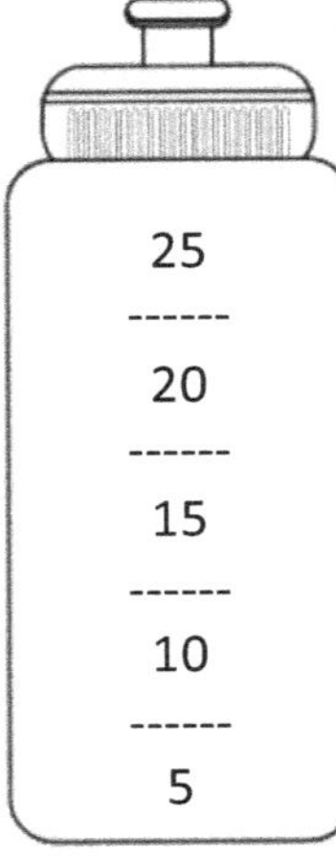

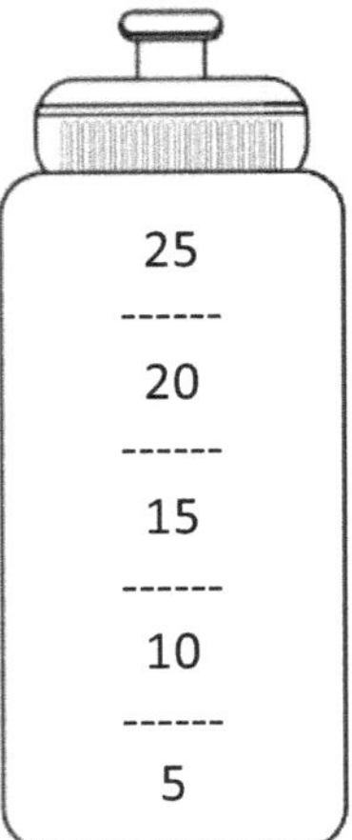

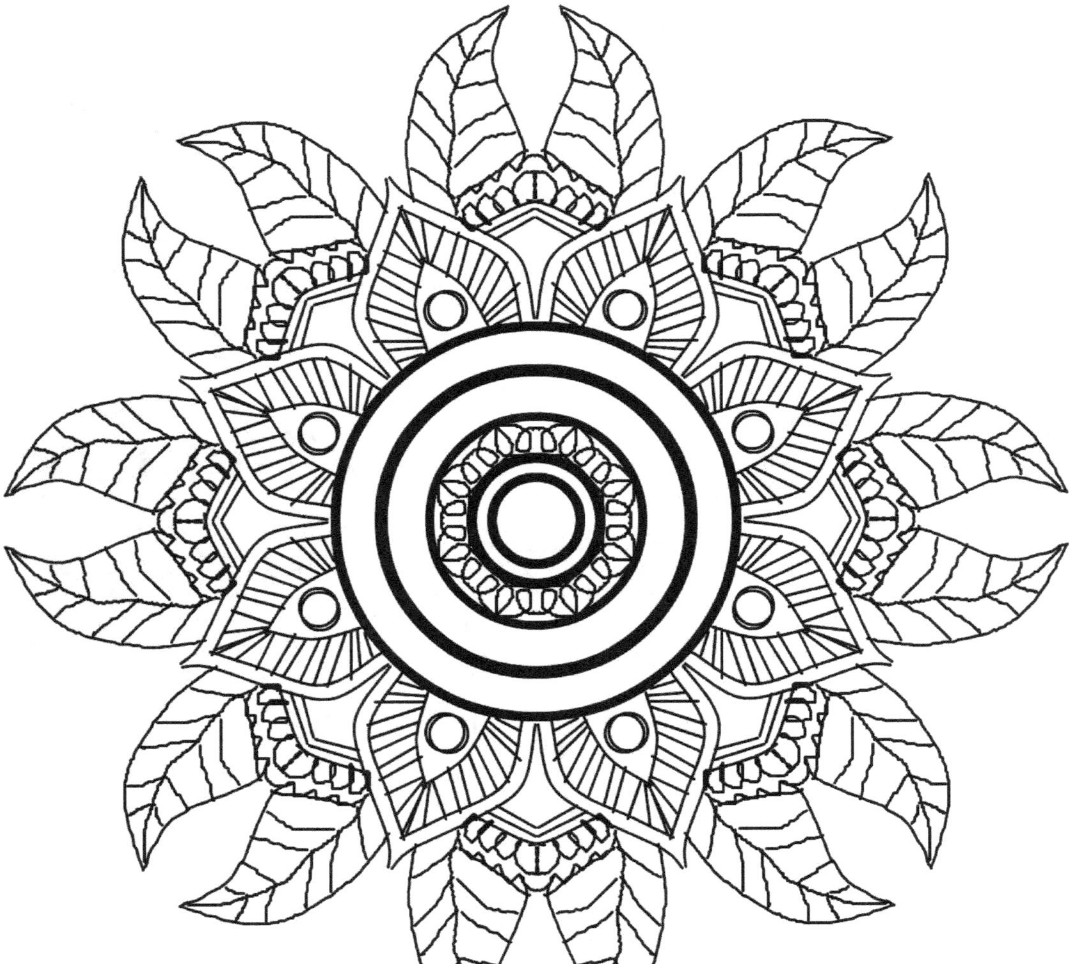

NOW WHAT?

www.ingramcontent.com/pod-product-compliance
Lightning Source LLC
Chambersburg PA
CBHW081612250726
48657CB00009B/2553
* 9 7 8 1 6 9 5 6 9 6 6 4 8 *